Bundles of Joy

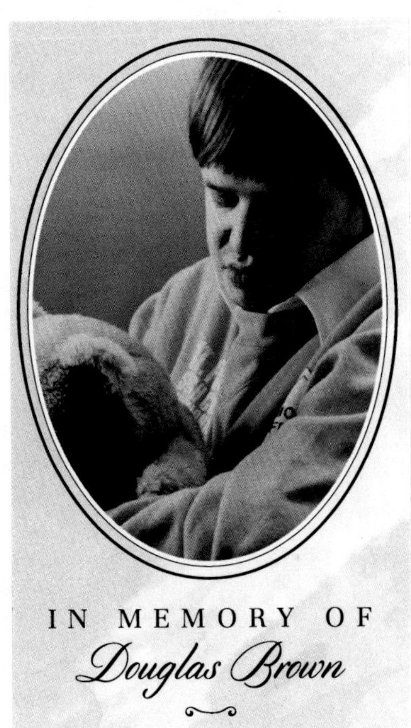

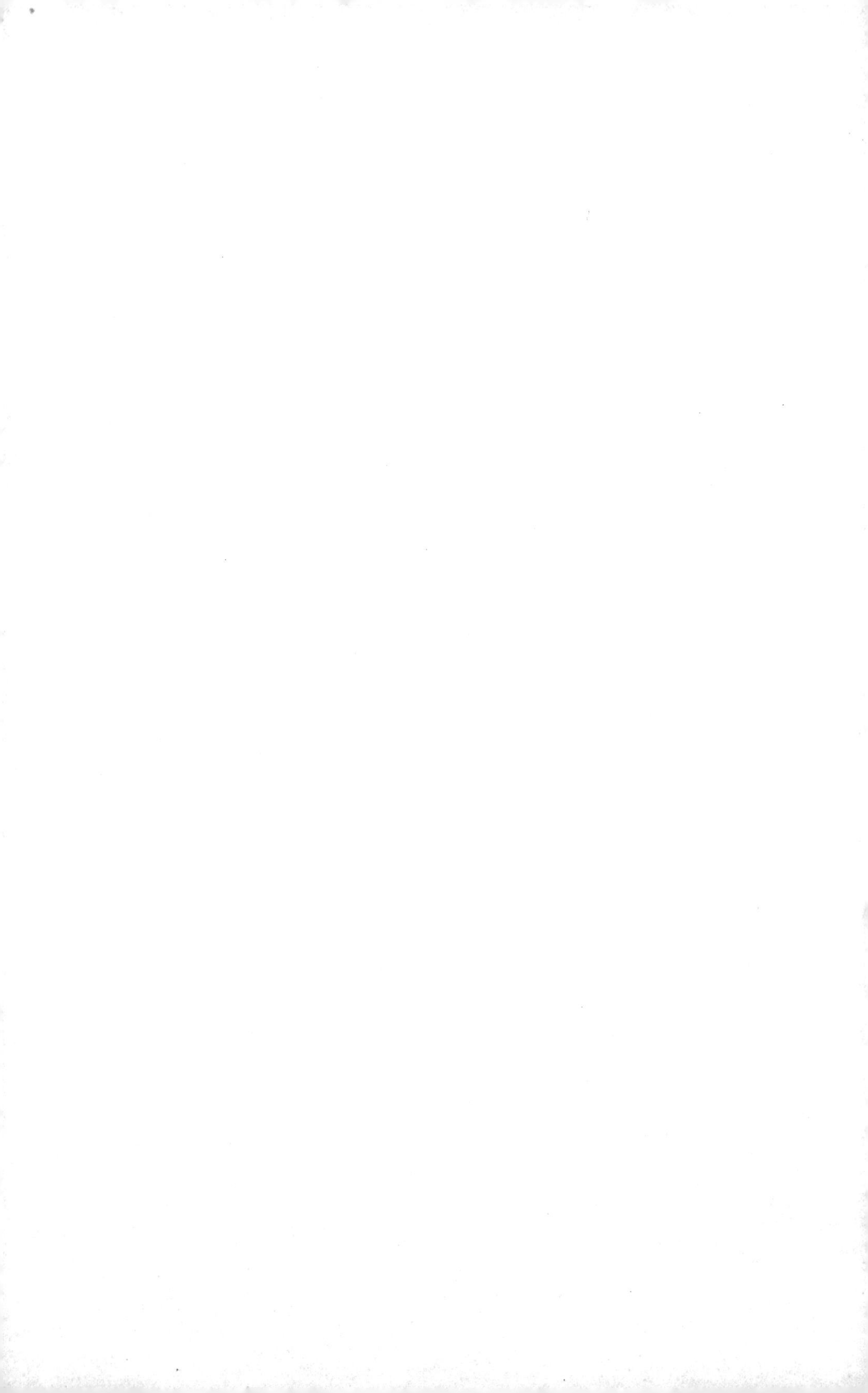

BUNDLES OF JOY

A JOURNEY BLESSED WITH TWO SPECIAL NEEDS CHILDREN

JANICE D. BROWN

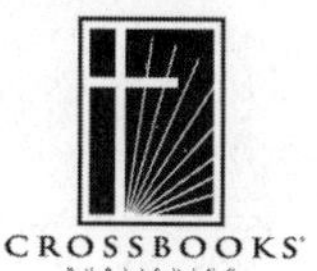

CrossBooks™
A Division of LifeWay
One LifeWay Plaza
Nashville, TN 37234
www.crossbooks.com
Phone: 1-866-768-9010

AU photo credit: Dennis Studio

First published by CrossBooks 06/20/2014

ISBN: 978-1-4141-2436-0 (sc)
ISBN: 978-1-4627-3730-7 (hc)
ISBN: 978-1-4627-3728-4 (e)

Library of Congress Control Number: 2014908671

Printed in the United States of America.

This book is printed on acid-free paper.

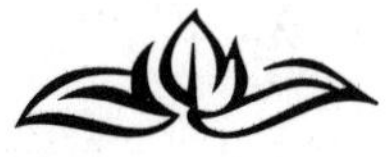

Dedicated

To my daughters, Lisa and Amy
My husband, Cowan
And to the memory of my son, Douglas

Contents

ACKNOWLEDGEMENTS

Thank you to my daughter, Lisa, who submitted text for the back cover, reading my early manuscript, and gave advice and help in remembering facts of years gone by.

Thank you to Mary Ellen Winner for being my sounding board and giving encouragement to get the job done. And, I appreciate your referral of an author to contact for publishing advice.

Thank you to Arlene Martin for time spent reading and rereading my manuscript, and for suggestions and encouragement.

Thanks and appreciation to Melmark Home for the love and care given to Douglas and Amy when Melmark became their home away from home.

My desire is that God will use this book to bring inspiration to others who may be in the throes of difficult times, using my experiences to show that He will give comfort, encouragement, and joy even through heartbreak, discouragement, frustration, and confusion.

Introduction

This book is a true account of joys and trying times I experienced as the mother of what I refer to as my "gifts": two severely, profoundly brain-damaged children—labeled as retarded. In today's society, "mentally challenged" would be the politically correct label for two of heaven's very special children, my bundles of joy. However, in the years of adventures with my children, the label that was relayed to me was indeed "retarded."

In this book, I present my children's diagnoses, messages, and reports in the same way they were presented to me. It all started when I was eagerly waiting for my first baby to arrive and to look forward to good times with him—the diagnosis was heartbreaking and difficult to understand. And then with the announcement of a second baby having the same diagnosis, confusion and frustration were added to my heartbreak. The joys I received, even in the midst of undesirable and distressing events, made the journey worthwhile.

In the movie *Forrest Gump*, Forrest says, "Life is like a box of chocolates. You never know what you're gonna get," and that would certainly describe my life journey. I know from the experience of selecting a piece of chocolate that I either will be given joy in the selection or an unpleasant experience I hope I never will face again. However, life does not give the opportunity to know what those "chocolates" will be in advance. I would have preferred my life to be like a box of Whitman's chocolates with labels that provide the opportunity to select only the good ones.

Many times I have had the pleasure of presenting a digest version of *Bundles of Joy* during speaking engagements, and was encouraged to write a book. The comments would be, you must have many more experiences with your children that you have not been able share in such a short time schedule. Yet I never considered myself an author, and so I dismissed the requests as something I never could do.

In recent years, the thoughts of recording the experiences with my special children kept coming to my mind but I continued to dismiss them as not being my cup of tea. However, about three years ago those thoughts became more pressing every Sunday during the church service. It seemed that either a part of the sermon or a song would say to me, "Write the book. Write the book." It eventually became apparent to me that a Higher Authority was, at that point, sending the "write the book" nudge and telling me the time is now.

Chapter 1

Two of my children could not walk, talk, or feed themselves and could not be toilet trained—and then my husband began to go blind. As I have traveled life's journey with these loved ones, I have walked the roads of love, joy, laughter, trial, and discouragement. Each of these roads, in its own way, has molded and shaped my character and personality and has made me who I am.

Maneuvering the mountain highs of love, joy, and laughter has given me great fulfillment, while the valley lows of trials and discouragement have given me strength in adversity. My challenging and sometimes heartbreaking conditions have been trying at times, but they have also helped make the steps of each mile a rewarding experience. I have been fortunate to have had the pleasure of understanding and supportive traveling companions, including family, friends, and acquaintances.

Many years ago an acquaintance asked, "How do you feel toward God because of the trials He has allowed into your life?" She was referring to the conditions I have faced as I have loved and cared for the Bundles of Joy that God gave me. That question caught me off guard because I had never had any feelings toward God but gratitude, both for the joyful *and* unpleasant circumstances that came into my life.

In a worship service one Sunday I heard the following illustration in a sermon by Dr. Stephen Hutchison. It describes my emotions—not specifically toward God but in general—as I was being molded and formed on the roads, mountains, and valleys.

A man and woman who were collectors of antiques and fine china were touring Sussex, England. As they passed a china shop, they stopped and went inside. There, their eyes singled out a teacup on a shelf.

He looked at her and said, "I have never seen a teacup like this one. It is beautiful."

The wife, excited about their find, agreed as she stared at the teacup.

Suddenly the teacup spoke and said, "You don't understand. I have not always been a teacup. There was a time when I was just a lump of clay. My master took me and rolled me and patted me again and again and again. I objected, 'Leave me alone!' He only smiled and said, 'Not yet.'"

Then the teacup said, "I was placed on a potter's wheel and was spun round and round and round. Again, I objected and said, 'Stop it! I am getting dizzy.' But the master only smiled and nodded and said, 'Not yet.'"

Then he put me in an oven. I had never felt so much heat! I wondered why he wanted to burn me up. I yelled and knocked at the door. I could see him through the opening and I could read his lips as he slowly shook his head and said, "Not yet.."

Finally, the door slid open, and he proudly took me out of the oven and carefully placed me on the shelf. I began to cool.

"Humpf!" I said. "That's better."

Then he started to brush and paint me all over. The fumes were horrible. I mean; I thought I would gag.

I cried out again, "Stop it! Stop it!"

But he only nodded and said, "Not yet..." Then, of all things, he put me back into the oven—not the first one, but an oven that was twice as hot. I knew I was going to suffocate. I begged; I pleaded, I cried. I knew there was no more hope and that I would never make it.

I was ready to give up, but then ... wait ... the door opened, and the master took me out of the oven and again placed me on the shelf. An hour later, he handed me a mirror and said, "Look at you."

I did and said, "That's not me. It couldn't be me. I-I-I'm beautiful!"

Then he said to me, "I know you remember how it hurt to be rolled and patted, but if I had left you the way you were, you would have dried up. I know the fumes were bad when I brushed and painted you all over, but as you see, if I had not done that, there never would have been any color in your life, and if I hadn't put you back in the second oven, you would not have survived very long. The fire gave you hardness and strength you wouldn't have had. Now, you are a finished product. You are what I had in mind when I first began, and now you can be useful to me."

That sermon illustration described the similarities between a teacup's "life" and feelings and the circumstances and feelings I had experienced and was experiencing even as I listened to the story. Pastor Steve is a good friend and he knew the circumstances in my life and the trials they had brought—the ones that caused people to ask about my feelings toward God. But, I do not know if he realized just how closely the teacup illustration aligned with my life.

I grew up in a Christian home where I was taught that God loved me and would always be available when I needed Him. I am thankful my parents took me to church and Sunday school every Sunday; because it was there that I got the foundation I would need later. At the age of eight I put my faith and trust in Jesus to be my Lord and Savior. At that time I had an understanding of what it meant to accept Him as Savior.

However, I only thought I understood what it meant to receive Him as Lord of my life. I had the head knowledge of His being my Lord, but it would be the circumstances a few years later that would teach me what it really meant to let Him be Lord in my everyday living.

During those childhood Sunday school years I heard many Bible stories, and was required to memorize Bible verses relating to those stories. I could not understand why memorizing Bible verses was so important. I thought it was a useless exercise. *Why should I memorize verses that I will probably forget?* Little did I know that those verses would be the glue that would hold me together in later years. If I had known then what life would bring on the roads, mountains, and valleys I walked later, I would have memorized and hidden more of them deep in my heart. It has been a wonder to me how many times those very verses came to mind at the exact time that I desperately needed their help and guidance. I have found the memory to be an amazing part of the brain—just waiting to be needed and used.

During the memory verse phase of my life, Cowan Brown was also participating in it at the same Sunday school and church. As time passed and we arrived at the junior high and high school years, we both joined the youth fellowship group at church. We enjoyed the companionship of other young people and participation in the youth group activities. As time went by, I began to notice Cowan and thought he was pretty cool.

Actually, I was aware he was pretty cool even before I became part of the youth group: at eleven years of age I had told my mother, "I am going to marry Cowan Brown." Since there was a four-year difference in our ages, she just laughed and said, "He does not even know you are alive." I told her, "He will." As time went on, Cowan did take notice (told you so, Mom!), and he and I paired up—as did others in the group—on Sunday outings. Eventually, Cowan and I began dating outside the youth group activities.

Upon graduating high school, Cowan enrolled in the University of Michigan's Navy ROTC program, and after graduation, he went on active duty in the Navy as an ensign, gave the next three years to Uncle Sam.

I had to wait a few years for our wedding day, but that was okay. I had college ahead of me at the University of Toledo. I was envious of Cowan, though, because while I was in school studying and waiting, he was aboard the USS Intrepid aircraft carrier, navigating the Mediterranean and seeing the beautiful and interesting places I had only dreamed about seeing someday. On one of his leaves, Cowan surprised me with a beautiful diamond engagement ring. Now I knew it was for real! There was going to be a wedding day. When his leave was over, he went back to his Navy assignment and I went back to studying, and started planning one of the most important days of my life—our wedding.

Chapter 2

As I awoke on March 2, 1957, my wedding day, my eyes were drawn toward my bedroom window. *Oh no,* I thought, *it's snowing. It's beautiful to look at the snow on the trees, fences, and housetops, but please, Lord, not on my wedding day.* By late afternoon, my prayer was answered. The snow stopped, and the sun began to shine.

As Mom and I were nervously buttoning my wedding gown, which she and I had designed and created, I asked her, "Mom, do you remember …" and before I could complete the rest of the question, she said, "Yes, I have been thinking about it all day." What I was about to ask her was if she remembered what I had told her when I was eleven years old—that someday I was going to marry Cowan Brown. And that was what I was doing that day—marrying Cowan Brown.

The weather presented Cowan and me with a beautiful evening for our wedding and reception. My heart filled with joy as I walked down the aisle on my father's arm, and as he placed my hand in Cowan's.

After receiving the congratulations and best wishes from our wedding guests at our reception, we left for our honeymoon in the Pocono Mountains. From the Poconos we traveled to Long Island, New York, not knowing where we were going to live, or even where we would sleep that night. I have thought many times over the years that if my daughter did that, I would be worried to death. New York of all places!

I grew up in Toledo, Ohio, which was a much smaller town than New York City, and had heard stories about what happens in the Big

Apple. But at that time I was blasé about those things, and knew I had a strong husband to protect me. I just knew my life would be perfect. Cowan was still in the Navy, stationed at St. Albans Naval Hospital, Long Island, New York, when we were married.

Not long before our wedding he had hip surgery to remove a benign tumor, and was still recovering from the surgery. Upon our arrival in New York, he checked into the hospital to have himself taken off leave. Even though he was still attached to the hospital, he was not required to reside in the hospital.

Since we did not have a place to live, we checked the message board at the hospital to find an apartment. There were no apartments available, but there was an ad for a room for rent with kitchen privileges. Since we had no other place to sleep that night, we made the call, and fortunately the room was still available. We rented it.

We knew right away that we were going to enjoy living there. The landlady was single and quite a character. Having kitchen privileges worked out well for all of us. I had her dinner ready when she came home from work, and I had the opportunity to test my culinary skills on my new husband. We had some laughs and good times telling stories about our lives and listening to hers. It seemed to be the best answer for her loneliness and our need of a place to live.

However, that perfect situation lasted only a short time. One day our landlady announced that she would be getting married soon and we would have to find another place to live, especially since the "one room" she had rented to us was the master bedroom. From our one-room living arrangement, we moved to a one-bedroom, third-floor, walk-up apartment in a private home. It was an interesting apartment that had originally been the attic. The walls were about four feet high and then angled steeply up to the ceilings, which were only about five feet wide. Cowan was more than six feet tall, so to keep from bumping his head he had to duck his head, and walk sideways while getting into bed. The walls and ceiling in the bedroom were brown beaverboard, and kind of depressing. If you know how rough beaverboard is, you know that Cowan really did not want to bump his head as he was getting into bed.

The rooms' depressing brown color finally started to cause us to feel depressed, and we asked the landlord if we could paint. We asked if she would purchase the paint. Hesitantly, she agreed. Our first experience of what it would be like if we ever had the opportunity to be homeowners was comical. We would roll a roller full of paint on the wall and by the time we had the roller filled with paint and turned back to continue, there was no paint on the wall, at least none that we could see. It had disappeared totally soaked in. Actually, you could hear it soaking in. It sounded like someone slurping a drink. So many coats of paint were needed to cover the beaverboard that we had to approach the landlord for more paint. She could not understand why we should need more, so we asked her to come and watch. She watched the paint disappear, and started laughing along with us. She agreed that we did need more paint. I am sure that that paint job ended up being more expensive than she had planned!

We had many laughs during those times in that apartment. Our bedroom was directly over the landlord's bedroom, and one night as we were getting into bed the slats holding the mattress and springs fell to the floor, along with the both of us, and made a very loud thud. We couldn't stop laughing at how ridiculous we must look, and we wondered what our landlords were thinking. It must have caused them to awaken with a jolt and sit up in bed.

The next morning she asked, "What on earth happened in the night? We heard such a loud noise." When we told her what had happened, she had a good laugh and said, "You are surely having some interesting experiences."

Cowan's recovery from hip surgery proceeded well, and when he was released from the hospital, we continued to enjoy happy and carefree lives together in our freshly-painted apartment. We enjoyed living in the area, but on an ensign's pay we were not able to take advantage of all the cultural and entertainment venues New York City had to offer. We saw the Empire State Building (from the sidewalk), and the Statue of Liberty (from the Staten Island Ferry). We did, however, ride the subway. It was a fascinating experience—I'm sure the wide-eyed look on my face, as the train went speeding through dark tunnels and flew past people waiting on platforms for their train; let everyone watching me know that I had never been on a subway.

After his release from the hospital, Cowan was assigned to the naval base in Bayonne, New Jersey. He spent most of his time traveling back and forth from Long Island to Bayonne, leaving home about 5 a.m. and returning around eight in the evening. This schedule was not the most conducive for a newly married couple, so we decided to move closer to the naval base. We found and rented an apartment close to the base.

There was another very important reason for moving: we found that we were going to become parents. With this news, we began to realize that Cowan should be closer as the time approached for our baby's birth, not 90 minutes away and having to depend on public transportation when "the time" came. We moved to Bayonne, about three blocks from the gate of the Navy post. We were young and naïve and thought that we had control of our lives as we waited for the birth of our baby—a baby that would add excitement to our perfect life.

Chapter 3

On October 15, 1958, our lives changed forever. Douglas, the baby we had been eagerly awaiting for nine months, was born at the US Public Health Hospital on Staten Island. He was our bundle of joy. What joy it was to hold this tiny little creature—this gift from God—and how proud we were.

When Douglas was placed in my arms for the first time, I thought, *here is a future president of the United States.* My heart filled with joy and wonder when I looked into the sweet, innocent face of this tiny little guy who had been a part of me. I marveled at such tiny fingers and toes. *My own could never have been as tiny! My skin could never have been as soft!* Each time the nurses brought him to feed, he had a fresh, clean smell of baby powder, and he looked handsome dressed in his little gown and wrapped in a soft, cuddly, blue baby blanket.

Of course, Dad was a proud papa. He had a boy! One day he was making his way down the corridor for a visit to see his bundle of joy, and when he arrived at the viewing window the nurse was waiting there holding up Douglas for him to see. Cowan said to her, "How did you know he was my baby?" She replied, "Well, he is, isn't he? You can't deny this is your child—he looks just like you." I am sure Dad started making mental plans of the father-son activities he and Doug would have as the baby grew through childhood and into adulthood.

In the 1950's, the hospital stay after giving birth was seven days, but it seemed twice that long to me. I was eager to go home and start having fun with my little bundle. Cowan and I were excited and proud as we brought our new little person home to join us in our apartment and to introduce him to our friends and neighbors. We were living many miles away from Toledo and our families, so they had to wait to meet him.

When we got past the excitement of the birth and congratulations of family and friends, it was time to move on to the reality of parenthood. *Now what do we do and how do we do it?* It did not take long to learn what and how things needed to be done. When he cried, feeding, changing, cuddling, rocking, singing, and walking the floor were the answers. As we went about the daily tasks of caring for our baby, it did not take long to find out that my sweet, fresh, clean, baby powder-smelling baby could have other smells too! I also found I had to be at attention at all times, and never turn my back on him.

One time while bathing Doug, he was lying on his back on the kitchen counter when I turned to grab a towel. When I turned back, to my shock I found he had turned from his back to his stomach! Of course, I knew this was going to happen sooner or later, but it still amazed me. I thought, *Wow, not only president, but a fast learner too!*

But then the excitement and fun we had anticipated enjoying when we brought Douglas home began to change. He cried day and night, and we found that the feeding, changing, rocking, cuddling, singing, and walking the floor were not working. I began to think he must have colic as I had heard happened with some babies. I also remembered hearing that burping would sometimes take care of that situation. So we added patting him on the back to our rocking and floor walking— but that didn't work either.

What happened to the fun and excitement I should have with my new baby? Motherhood had turned into chores and frustration. It was frustrating not being able to find a way to comfort and console him, and it became a chore because most of my day was filled with these consoling and comforting efforts.

When Cowan came home from work, I was more than ready to turn the rocking, cuddling, patting on the back, and walking the floor over to him. As we spent our days and nights walking, I remembered another comment I had heard—that babies sometimes get their days and nights mixed up. They sleep in the daytime and are awake at night. Well that certainly was happening at our house. However, the crying was not only at night. It was day and night!

There were five other families living in the apartment house, plus our landlord's family. What a predicament! We had to find a way to keep Doug quiet, at least at night, but nothing seemed to help. One time in the middle of the night, the crying was so intense that while I was trying to find a way to quiet him, I thought, *if you do not stop crying I am going to throw you against the wall.* Very quickly I said, "Oh, Lord, forgive me. Please give me patience." I immediately felt shame, but at the same time I thought something similar to that must be what happens when we hear on the news that a baby is abused in such a manner. I woke Cowan and asked him to take over for a while. I needed a break, and some sleep—if that was possible.

I am sure I was sleep deprived most of the time during those days. I remember feeling drained and very tired. Many times while I was trying to feed Doug during the night I was sleepy and nodding off. I would hear the bottle hit the floor and feel Doug slipping out of my arms in that direction. The noise of the bottle hitting the floor would cause me to sit straight up at attention.

Several weeks went by, and it was time for Doug's newborn follow-up visit with the pediatrician. I poured out my frustration with the constant crying to the doctor. His first comment was, just as I had been thinking, "He probably has colic." However, while he was examining Douglas, he said, "No, I don't think it is colic. I may have found a reason for the excessive crying." He discovered double hernias in our little guy, one on each side. He said the crying might be caused by the pain from the hernias and/or may have caused the hernias to appear. Surgery would probably be in Doug's future.

"Surgery? I said, "On such a tiny person? Can that be done? Should it be done?" The doctor said, "That may be our only solution." In the meantime, he suggested raising the foot of the crib to relieve pressure in the hope that the hernias would eventually subside and possibly disappear. His hope was that raising the bed would at least lessen the pain and stop some of the crying.

We followed the doctor's advice and raised the crib, but that did not work either. We continued to walk, rock, cuddle, and sing. We discovered that rides in the car sometimes would put him to sleep. We were fairly new residents in the Bayonne area at the time, but we did not stay strangers to the geography and area sights very long. We spent many hours riding around, hoping for peace and quiet. The outings to lull Doug to sleep took us to new places and we took advantage of his sleeping, if that happened, to continue checking the sights.

Even though these rides sometimes would put Doug to sleep, they did not do much to help our exhaustion and sleep deprivation. Since all efforts to deal with the hernias had failed, when Doug was five weeks old the doctors decided to do surgery.

Cowan and I had some apprehensions. As we had wondered earlier, could this be done—and should it be done—on a baby? We knew something had to be done to prevent the pain. We had done all we could do. At that point, all we knew to do was turn this situation over to the Lord. We did not know what else to do.

As the day for the surgery approached; we prayed for God to give guidance, wisdom, and skill to the doctor for Doug's safe and successful surgery. We called family and friends and requested they join us in prayer. Even though I had questioned if surgery was feasible on a baby, I do not remember feeling anxiety at the fact that my tiny five-week-old bundle of joy was about to undergo a serious violation of his fragile little body.

As I think back, I do not recall anxious moments even during the surgery. I am not sure if it was naivety that gave me the sense of calm, or complete trust in knowing God was in control and was watching over Doug as we had asked Him to do. The US Public Health Service Hospital where the surgery was performed did not have a pediatric division, so mother, was required to check into the hospital room with her baby, and be the caregiver day and night for everything except administering medications.

The operation to repair both hernias was scheduled for 8 a.m. During the operation on the first hernia, the doctor said something caused him to think perhaps Doug could not make it through an operation on both sides. So the decision was made to repair only one side and leave the other side to be done at a later date. My bundle of joy was brought back to his room, and then it was my job to watch, change, and feed.

As I watched and waited, I thanked God for bringing him through the surgery. The minutes seemed like hours as I patiently watched and waited for my job to begin. Since it was my responsibility to care for his needs, I checked every few minutes, watching for signs of rousing. As the hours passed I became concerned that Douglas was not waking or showing signs of life.

Many times I mentioned my concern to the nurses, only to be told that he was okay. They said, "He's a tiny baby, and it will take time for the anesthesia to wear off." I could hear the condescension in their voices: "You are a young mother. What do you know about giving nursing care to sick people?"

I was aware of the fact that the anesthesia would take time to wear off, but I felt it should be happening by that time. I was also aware that I was a young mother, and definitely did not know about nursing sick people in the professional, medical manner the staff did. But, I also knew that my bundle of joy had just been through a traumatic experience, and it seemed to me that, after all the hours of watching and waiting, he should be waking.

By late afternoon I became very uneasy and demanded that the nurses do a more thorough check on Doug, or I would call the doctor and request that he come and check. My instincts told me something was wrong.

Begrudgingly, the nurse came into the room, turned on better lighting, and immediately said to me, "Go to the lobby and wait. We will call you when we know what is happening." She left the room, running down the hallway calling for help, "STAT!" I felt a sharp stab in my heart that took my breath away because I knew that "STAT" meant trouble. I am sure the nurse finally saw what had been my concern for about four or five hours. The reason I had been "bugging" her was that my baby was as white as the sheet he was lying on, his fingernails were turning blue, and he was not responding to my touches.

I dutifully did as I was told; I went trembling to the lobby to wait. The wait in the empty lobby seemed to be hours long, and the naivety that I'd had before the surgery was now turning to fear and anxiety. Cowan could not be with me during the surgery because he had command duty of the ship. However, when I got that reaction from the nursing staff, I called him to come. I really needed him to be there for comfort and support. He found a replacement to take over his command and arrived to wait with me.

The nursing staff called the doctor to assess the situation. When he arrived, he told us he didn't know what the problem was but that he would examine Doug and then let us know. The hours of waiting started to feel like an eternity, but we knew what to do while waiting—we prayed, "God, You gave us this baby to love and care for. Please help the doctor find and resolve the problem."

Finally, calm came as we continued to wait to hear the doctor's report. After the examination, the doctor came to tell us they had discovered blood in the scrotum and would have to reopen his tiny body and find out what was going on. He thought perhaps the inside sutures were not holding.

When the incision was reopened, the doctor found all the previous work was perfect, but with each heartbeat there was internal hemorrhaging. Tests showed that the bleeding was caused by his body not processing Vitamin K, which produces fibrinogen that is critical for blood clotting. By that time, Doug had lost a large portion of his blood and needed a transfusion to replace it. He was so small and his veins so tiny that the technicians could not locate a vein they could use to start the transfusion. They tried to insert a needle into every vein they thought might work on his hands, arms, legs, and elsewhere on his body. Finally, a cut down in the ankle provided access for a tube to be inserted into the vein. This was all, finally, accomplished at one a.m.—seventeen hours and two surgeries later.

As soon as the doctor felt the situation was under control, we were allowed to see Doug. I felt very relieved as I looked at the rosy color that had returned to his body. This was what I had been waiting to see after the first surgery.

From that point, the recovery time proceeded as expected while I did my "nursing" job. We thanked God for guiding the surgeon's decision to repair only one hernia. Had he done both, Doug might not have survived. We thanked God for watching over Doug and answering our prayers for successful surgeries.

A few more days went by while I carried out my "nursing" and mothering role. Then it was time to bring Doug home. Now our family could be happy forever after, I thought. How wonderful it was going to be to enjoy our baby without the constant crying! Our apartment was now finally quieter, and Doug seemed to be comfortable. I am sure the landlord and the other tenants also appreciated the quietness. We knew we still had the second hernia surgery coming soon, but for the time being we could relax and return to living a normal life.

Chapter 4

During a routine follow-up visit to the doctor to have Doug's incision area checked, the doctor became concerned that his development seemed to be slow.

"But we do have to remember that he has been through a lot for a tiny baby," he said.

We had also noticed that Doug was not doing some of the things he had done before the surgery, such as turning over from back to stomach, as he had displayed while I was bathing him during the first weeks after his birth. This was our first experience at parenting, though, so we thought maybe this was not unusual—but after the doctor's comments about slow development; we began to have concerns ourselves.

Realizing I could not go through another recovery period of taking care of Doug in the US Public Hospital, both the doctors and Cowan and I decided that, for the second surgery, we would take him to a hospital that could provide pediatric recovery nursing care. This was a great relief for me because I had been dreading going through that experience again. I knew what had happened was not my fault, but I also knew I would feel more comfortable with professionals being the responsible care givers.

Plans were made for him to be admitted to Saint Albans Naval Hospital, the hospital where his dad had had his hip surgery.

The second hernia surgery went well with no complications. Precautions were taken before this surgery to assure that there would be no hemorrhaging this time. While Doug was in the hospital for this surgery, a neurological survey of his brain determined why his development seemed to be going so slowly. The results of the tests were that he had genetic brain damage.

Due to the doctors feeling it was a genetic situation, we were told we should have no more children. I could not believe what I had just heard! As I listened to those words, it felt like my whole body was turning to gelatin. I was wobbly and unstable. When I finally regained some semblance of composure, I asked God what was happening and to please take control of this situation and let it not be so. I felt any dreams I had for Doug were slipping away, especially those I had the day he was born—that one day he would be the president.

I began to understand that sometimes my best hopes and dreams might be shattered by events over which I had no control. This event was definitely the beginning of the shattering of the hopes and dreams for my bundle of joy, but it was also the beginning of a long and beautiful relationship with God, who did have control over all things in our lives.

The diagnosis news began to travel over the miles to family and friends. Soon phone calls, cards, and notes began to arrive, bringing messages of comfort and support. One of the notes included a poem that deeply touched my heart, and that has become a treasure to my life. This same poem has been given to me several other times over the years as other incidents, which I share later in this book, occurred. The title of the poem is "Heaven's Very Special Child." Most mothers have had the same thrill and opportunity I had of holding their newborn babies. However, not many may have had the opportunity of experiencing the special kind of joy I have because of my "special child."

The question may be asked, "Aren't all children special?" Yes, all children are special, but this poem describes my "special child."

Heaven's Very Special Child

A meeting was held quite far from earth
"It's time again for another birth,"
Said the Angels to the Lord above,
"This special child will need much love."

His progress may seem very slow,
Accomplishments he may not show,
And he'll require extra care
From folks he meets down there.

He may not run or laugh or play;
His thoughts may seem quite far away.
In many ways he won't adapt,
And he'll be known as handicapped.

So let's be careful where he's sent.
We want his life to be content.
Please, Lord, find the right parents who
Will do this special job for You.

They will not realize right away
The leading role they're asked to play.
But with this child sent from above
Comes stronger faith and richer love.

And soon they'll know the privilege given
In caring for this gift from heaven.
Their precious charge, so meek and mild
Is heaven's very special child.

By Edna Massimilla
Hatboro, PA 19040
(Reprinted with permission)

Each time I have received and reread this poem it reminds me of Psalm 139:13-14: "For you created my inmost being; you knit me together in my mother's womb. I praise you because I am fearfully and wonderfully made; your works are wonderful, I know that full well." These were verses I memorized many years ago in my early Sunday school days.

While Doug was hospitalized for the second surgery, we asked a friend from church—a navy doctor and ophthalmologist at Saint Albans Naval Hospital—to see if he could get information about what had happened during Doug's first surgery. In our discussions with him, we began to wonder if during that first surgery the blood tests usually done before surgery had been done properly or even at all; and if so, were the results properly read. Proper testing should have shown there was going to be a problem before the surgery, and steps could have been taken that would have prevented the hemorrhaging. Our friend did extensive searching but was unable to find answers. While examining Doug, our doctor friend suspected Doug also had a vision problem. He said Doug's retinas looked like salt and pepper, which was not normal.

Even though our friend tried to comfort Cowan and me, and to turn our thoughts and concerns toward positive thoughts, I was beginning to feel defeated and helpless. I had always been in control of most situations in my life, but now it seemed there was nothing I could do to control this one, and it was exasperating. All my life I had been taught that God, the creator, has the power over all He has created and He has the power to move mountains. I was certainly thankful for Doug, this gift He had created within me, and I prayed, "Here is a mountain, Lord. Please, please move it. I know you have the power to do all things, because all things belong to you, and I trust you will do this."

As my mind ran rampant with questions, I was trying to have the faith of that mustard seed I had read about in Sunday school, the verse that says, "Truly I tell you, if you have faith as small as a mustard seed, you can say to this mountain, 'Move from here to there,' and it will move" (Matthew 17:20). Well, I didn't want to mess up moving such an important mountain as this myself, so with faith, I turned over moving this mountain to God's power. I tried to let the knowledge that He has control over these circumstances be comforting, but there was still a side of me that was worried, uneasy, and anxious. But I have always had a spirit of persistence when it comes to overcoming obstacles, and I did not intend to give up on this obstacle without persistently asking for God's intervention.

While I was feeling the hurt and frustration, a quiet voice from within said, "Let your life be content with such things as you have. I will never leave you or forsake you,"

I prayed, "Yes, I know, Lord, that you say to 'be content with what I have, and that you will never leave or forsake me' that is why I am putting my trust in you to remove this 'mountain' from Douglas."

Again and again, the quiet voice said, "I will never allow a burden that you cannot bear."

I wondered why "a burden you cannot bear" kept coming to my attention. Another puzzling part of the verse that kept repeating in my mind was "and be content with what you have." *Content with what I have!* Now I was beginning to get a feeling I did not like, one that made me very uncomfortable. Was being "content with what you have" the Lord's way of telling me this is the way it will be? Well, maybe, but if this was truly what was to be, I could not give up without asking and even pleading before accepting.

Chapter 5

Cowan's tour of active duty with the Navy was nearing an end, and we started making plans for our move back to Ohio. Doug was about four months old at the time of the move. During the consultation at Doug's release from the hospital, the doctors suggested that, near Doug's first birthday, we have the neurological tests repeated for comparison, and to determine the extent of the neurological problem.

We finally had the opportunity to introduce our bundle of joy to our family and friends, and settled back into our hometown's familiar surroundings. Cowan began his chemical engineering career with Sun Oil Company and joined the Navy Reserve, and I resumed being a happy homemaker, wife, and mother. Doug's situation was definitely not normal compared to that of most babies, so I thought it would be a good idea to take him to visit the pediatrician before he became ill so the doctor could see and understand what his "normal" life was.

That first visit to Dr. Baehren was definitely not what I was expecting. As he was examining Doug, he kept saying, kind of under his breath, "Hmm … mmm … mmm." I could tell by those sounds, and his demeanor, that he was concerned. After the exam, he asked me to dress Doug and come into his office; he needed to talk with me. As I was dressing Doug, the words the doctor said—"I need to talk with you"—triggered puzzling thoughts in my mind.

When I entered his office, the doctor was sitting with his hands cradling his chin, staring at an open file folder on his desk, and shaking his head in disbelief. With a look of concern on his face, and with a voice of compassion, he said, "I have never seen a child like this. When the cards were dealt, you got the worst hand I have ever seen. The only advice I can give you is to take him home and make him comfortable as long as you have him."

Hey, wait a minute, I thought. I did not expect a comment like this at a well-baby visit. I could sense the unstable feeling coming again—the one I had when we were told that Doug was brain damaged. I felt wobbly. Since this visit was for the doctor's information purposes only, Cowan had not gone with us. But with this blow, it certainly would have been comforting to have his company and support.

I asked the doctor, "What do you mean?"

His reply: "This child is so deeply involved; his heart will not be able to hold on very long."

Drawing a deep breath to give me the support, I needed to prepare me to hear what he would say, I asked, "How long is not very long?"

He replied, "About a year or so."

"Do you mean he will die?" I asked.

This thought had not crossed my mind. Douglas dying!

No, surely that would not happen. There had to be an answer to this situation. Again I prayed, "Lord, you gave Douglas to us, and you brought him through the surgeries. Surely you would not allow him to be taken away. Please, I am pleading again for your intervention. Let us know what we can do."

Several months passed by, during which Doug was healthy and did not need to visit Dr. Baehren. Then it was time to make an appointment for the one-year neurological testing that had been recommended in New York. Doug was admitted to the hospital for the tests, and we were asked to wait for Dr. Baehren to check on Doug and discuss the testing with us.

When the doctor arrived, he stopped by the room where we were waiting to say hello, and asked in which room he could find Doug. We told him the room number. He said, "I was just in that room, and I did not see him."

We went back to the room with him and pointed to Doug. He was amazed because he could not believe Doug was the same child he had seen a few months earlier.

He said, "I never thought I would see Doug alive for his first birthday and these tests, and definitely not in the condition I'm witnessing."

Cowan's sister, Rachel, and Dr. Baehren had been high school classmates. Their class had annual reunions. He and Rachel attended each year. He would ask her every year how Doug was doing, and each year the answer was, "Doing fine." After many years of the reunions, he said, "I will never tell parents anything like I told the Browns. I never expected Doug to live to be one year old. He has certainly made a liar out of me. It has to be the love and care he has been given, because if the Browns had taken my advice and placed him in an institution, he would have never lived this long."

The question became an annual occurrence, and Rachel said almost a joke. Their eyes would meet, even across the banquet room, and Dr. Baehren's expression would indicate, "Well, is Doug still living?" Rachel would nod her head yes. He would walk away, shaking his head in amazement—and probably "Hmmm, hmm-ing" as he had the first day he met and examined Doug at five months of age.

After years of this annual "questioning," Dr. Baehren passed away. He never knew how many years past that one-year prediction Doug survived—thirty-five years, to be exact.

Following that series of tests performed on one-year-old Doug and after the comparisons had been made to the New York tests, we were asked to come to the doctor's office for a consultation to review the results. I had put my trust in God, and my hopes and prayers were for results that would be different from those in New York. But, I could tell by the look on his face, as we entered the doctor's office that it probably was not good news, and it was not.

The results were the same as in New York. Brain damage, but this time the diagnosis was labeled "severely and profoundly brain damaged—retarded." *Retarded?* I could not believe what I was hearing. This report with the same results as the one in New York seemed to be destroying all hope of Doug's life being normal. The word "retarded" caused a storm to begin thundering in the deepest part of my being. I felt as if I were in the middle of a violent storm with thunder, lightning, and torrential rain all working together to tear me apart. I was trying to get a grip on the haunting thoughts I was having at hearing the word "retarded" being associated with my baby.

Then the doctor made a suggestion that gave me a real jolt. "Start looking for an institution," he said, "because Doug will be barely more than a vegetable." *Oh, no! Is there going to be no end to this? It's going from bad to worse!* Our immediate response was that an institution was not the answer. The thought of an institution made me uncomfortable because the picture that came to mind was a lonely place far away with strange looking and strange acting people. No, my cute, sweet baby was not going to a place like that.

We told Dr. Baehren that we would never consider that as an option unless it became necessary because of physical health or emotional problems, or if the situation affected other children in the family. Douglas had been given to our family. Our home was where God had placed him to be loved and given tender care.

With so many thoughts for my mind to grapple with, we took our bundle of joy home and began to deal with the manifestations that went with severely and profound brain damaged: retarded, not toilet trainable, not able to talk, not able to walk, not able to feed himself, and having serious vision problems. He was helpless!

Even though all these things were Doug's life at that point, he was a very happy and contented child. As I performed my motherly duties of caring for him, I had vivid memories of the day and night crying when he came into this world, and I was constantly grateful that he, or we, did not have to face that any longer.

I have to be honest—I was very grateful that I did not have to be faced with the task of cuddling, walking the floor, rocking, and singing in an attempt to comfort him to stop the crying. Instead, I could now do those things because he and I both enjoyed them, and it gave great comfort to both of us. I accepted the responsibilities of loving and caring for Douglas and his handicaps, but I could not give up my pleading for God to give alternatives.

Chapter 6

In 1960, when Doug was about two years old, we decided it was time for us to own a home of our own. We purchased a great little house and for the next couple years we made it our home. Douglas loved to swing in a tripod baby swing we had received as a baby shower gift. That swing gave him so much enjoyment that we installed a baby swing hanging from the ceiling on our new home's front porch. He would swing for hours while making his humming sounds of contentment. Doug wore out the toes of several pairs of shoes, pushing and dragging his feet as he swung.

Several children in the neighborhood were fascinated with Douglas. They would spend time on the porch with him while he was swinging. They would talk to him and did not seem to be concerned that he did not answer back or in any way acknowledge that he heard; they found out if they made loud noises, such as banging on the floor of the porch, Doug would laugh. Sometimes he would laugh so hard you would think he was going to fall out of the swing. The first time I heard the loud bang they made, I went running because I thought Doug had fallen out of the swing, but I found him and the children laughing. They would wait for Doug to relax and breathe a big sigh, and bang again and again. It gave me great pleasure to watch Doug and his "friends" having a good time laughing together. They kept him company, and he amused them.

The mothers of these children thanked me for sharing Doug with their children. They said their kids thought Doug was great, and they had fun playing with him. On the days, Doug was not swinging on the porch there would be a knock at the door and the little guys would ask if he could come out and play. It was thrilling to see and hear these children consider Doug a playmate rather than someone strange who would not talk to them and who seemed different from them. It was also amazing to me that they never asked questions. They just accepted.

Since he could not walk and had never learned to crawl, Doug started scooting around the house on his backside. He would cruise through the house at breakneck speed, his blindness not a hindrance. He could beat our walking from one room to another by scooting! We, and our friends were always amazed watching him. They would be very concerned as they observed him maneuver into the kitchen and head toward the stairway going down to the basement. They would gasp and lunge for the doorway. Our comment would be, "Wait, just watch." We never kept the door to the basement closed because we knew what was going to happen. He would scoot to the steps, and when he felt the heel of his foot drop over the top of the first step, turn on a dime and head back in the other direction, never missing a beat of the scooting motion.

Doug had never fallen down the stairs. How would someone with his severity of brain damage know not to go farther? He had never had the experience of falling down the steps, so that didn't explain it. There seemed to be some form of understanding there, and our prayers began to be that we could find what could be done to unlock this understanding, and then learn how to work with it to bring a better life for Doug. It was fun to watch these exercises, but at the same time, it was a confusing mystery.

Douglas was a mystery in many ways. There was a period of time when we had to have him wear a boxing glove. We never knew why, but he would bang his forehead and bridge of his nose with his fist until it bled. We tried everything we could think of to stop this activity, but nothing worked. Our greatest concern was that the open wound would become infected and cause serious problems. Fortunately that never happened. We consulted a doctor and asked if he had any suggestions as to why the head banging was happening and how to stop it. He jokingly said, "No, but if he wants to be a boxer, put boxing gloves on him."

We laughed along with the doctor, but I thought, *never considered that idea, but nothing else has worked so why not try?* To our surprise—it worked. He would still bang his head occasionally, but there would be no bleeding. However, he did end up with a black eye a few times. Try and explain that to your family, friends, and neighbors as you watch their puzzled looks and raised eyebrows! Still, we were frustrated that we couldn't understand why he banged his head. Was it just something to do to pass the time? Was he bored? Was he in pain?

The boxing glove was never laced and tied. He could have taken it off any time he chose, but he very rarely did. Some children have security blankets, and I suppose the boxing glove was his "security blanket." He wore the glove off and on for several weeks at a time. Time would pass by when he did not need it, and then back on it would have to go again for several weeks. This boxing glove scene went on four to five years. Then for some reason, which we never could figure out, it stopped—never to happen again.

Douglas was a picky eater in his early years. I remember so well the only two foods he would eat for four years: oatmeal for breakfast and Gerber split pea and bacon baby food for lunch and dinner—every day! Feeding him during those years was a chore for me because I had a serious dislike for split pea, even the smell. And the split pea and bacon baby food had to be Gerber brand, or he would not eat it. On many occasions, we tried other brands. Forget it—he would not eat it! Another puzzling part of Doug's life.

We were planning a trip to Florida and I became concerned about the possibility of not finding Gerber brand baby food for him. I had horrible thoughts that we would get to Florida and not find the Gerber brand, and he wouldn't eat—and then what would we do? Since we were driving, we couldn't just hop back on a plane for a fast trip home to "Gerberland" and his favorite food. We bought three cases to put in the trunk of the car--just to be safe.

Even though Doug could not see, his hearing was very acute. Noises were amusing to him. Whenever a semi would pass us in a tunnel going the opposite direction, the car would jump, and the noise would send Doug into spells of laughter. He would catch his breath and wait until he heard another truck coming in the distance, and then start chuckling. When the semi passed us, his laughing would become louder. If a trucker blew his horn for some reason, watching Doug just about choke while laughing so hard would send Cowan and me into such laughter that tears would flow.

Chapter 7

When Doug was around five years old, we started to discuss the feasibility of having another child. There were hours of discussion and prayer while seeking guidance and direction. My obstetrician knew Doug, and he knew that we had been told not to have other children and our apprehensions because of that advice. He told us the decision to add to our family should not be a concern. However, he was concerned about my picking up Douglas from the playpen or off the floor, and carrying him during a pregnancy, especially up and down stairs.

He said, "Let's take no chances and take every precaution we can" and suggested that when and if a sister or brother for Doug happened, we install a stair glide to at least take care of climbing the stairs with Doug.

(I later became aware that the stair chair glide was great for other functions, as well. It was handy to send the laundry and many other things up and down the stairs. And of course our friends' children thought it was a great plaything!)

I soon learned that I was pregnant. Then the questioning thoughts began creeping into my mind. *What have we done? Is this wise?* However, the pregnancy went well as we eagerly and anxiously awaited the blessing of the birth. On August 26, 1964, Lisa, our second bundle of joy, arrived. When the nurse gave her to me to hold for the first time, I quickly counted fingers and toes. *All here!* I checked every inch of her body to see if I could detect any abnormalities. My antennae were ready to pick up anything I might identify that would indicate a problem. If one occurred, I was ready to attack it right away. There did not seem to be any problems that I could see.

I remembered the cuddly blue blanket in which Doug was wrapped when I first saw him and my thoughts, *here is a future president.* Now looking at this cuddly little pink bundle, I thought, *She will be Miss America someday, or maybe the first female president.*

She also smelled of baby powder, and like Doug, had soft, soft skin and tiny fingers and toes. Since I found nothing to make my antennae perk up, I breathed a sigh of relief, but at the same time I thought, *there were no noticeable problems with Doug when I first held him either.* I had to reverse my thoughts from thinking negatively and remember God had given me this precious baby to love and enjoy—and that was what I was going to do.

What a joy it was to watch such a different development in this infant and child as she grew and matured! Unlike Doug's slow development that had concerned doctors, Lisa's development pleased the pediatrician, so that pleased me. She was an alert and precocious child. We were thankful for this blessing because it seemed apparent that there was no genetic situation to overshadow our family.

Activities around our house were now a little more time consuming, but at least we did not have a baby who cried constantly this time around. We were able to enjoy our cute, little, pink bundle of joy from the very first day.

The time soon came for Lisa's newborn baby follow-up appointment with the pediatrician. He announced we had a perfect baby, but again brought up the subject of an institution for Doug.

"For Lisa's sake," he said.

Again the answer was no. Both of these children belonged to God, and He had placed them in our care. The Lord had given us Douglas and we knew God made no mistakes. There had to be a reason, and we needed to wait for the answer from Him.

Chapter 8

Cowan arrived home from work one day with news—good or bad; I wasn't sure. Sun Oil was transferring him to Philadelphia. At this point, Douglas was five years old, and Lisa was six weeks. There was a part of me that was excited. We would have new experiences to enjoy and new people to meet. The other part of me thought; *I will be far away from our families who have been a great help with Doug and Lisa*. Yet I realized this move could offer advantages for Cowan's career, giving him the opportunity to "advance up the ladder."

The assignment was to be for one year. That wouldn't be too difficult to deal with, and then I could come back to family and help! Finally, the positive side of me won the battle, and we started making plans for the move.

The move to Philadelphia was accomplished in October. Soon snow started falling with an accumulation of about four inches on the ground. It was beautiful to see— clean and white. When the sun shone on the trees, they looked as if they were covered with sparkling diamonds.

Soon after the move, Cowan said he could not understand why he had been transferred. There did not seem to be a reason. The job was not special and anyone else could do it, he said. It also seemed strange that the company would take on the expense of moving us for a one-year assignment and then move us back to Toledo.

One morning, shortly after the move, Cowan left for work. Doug became restless and fussy. I put him in bed with me to keep him from waking Lisa, and we both went back to sleep. Soon I was awakened by the bed shaking and Doug making strange noises. His body was shaking. I turned him over to face me and with horror I realized he was having a seizure. That was the first time I had seen a seizure, but it seemed to match what I had read about them. It was scary, especially watching my own child acting so strangely.

I panicked. What was I to do? I knew I needed to get him to the hospital, but what about Lisa? Furthermore, I didn't see how I could drive in the snowy weather with my seizing child beside me. Then another thought came to mind. *There are four inches of snow on the driveway, and it is still snowing. How long will it take me to shovel away enough snow so I can even get the car out of the garage?*

I knew time was of the essence, and my panic was increasing as I paced the floor trying to decide what to do. I was in such a state that I didn't even think to call 911 for help. I finally decided to call a neighbor and tell her my problem. She suggested that I call the police. They would take Doug and me to the hospital, and she would come and stay with Lisa.

At the hospital emergency room, it was determined that Doug had a very high fever. He was immediately wrapped in an ice blanket to bring down the fever quickly. What screaming and crying he gave off at the shock of the cold blanket! Of course, he did not understand what was happening, and I could imagine it made him very uncomfortable. I was told that he was probably coming down with a cold or a respiratory infection, and the warmth of my body against his made his temperature shoot up, which had caused the seizure. It was important to bring his fever down immediately.

I stored the picture of Doug having the seizure in my memory bank so I would know what was happening next time—if there was to be a next time.

Doug was prone to upper respiratory infections. On another occasion, he came down with a cold that required a doctor visit. The visit was the first since we had moved, so it was this doctor's first meeting with Doug.

When the pediatrician finished examining him, he said to me, "What are you doing for Douglas?" Stunned, I ask what he meant. He said, "What are you doing to help Doug with his problems?" Of course, I had done nothing, other than love and care for him because I had been told it was a hopeless situation.

He said, "That might be true, but let me recommend a neurosurgeon, Dr. Eugene Spitz, who might be able to help you. He has had remarkable results with patients with brain damage situations."

My eyes lit up, and my heart and head started to pound at the thought that there might be help for Doug. My heart was telling me to get excited, but my head was telling me, *Hold on, don't get too excited. It might not work.* As the days went by and we waited for an appointment with this new doctor, my mind could not help becoming enthusiastic. Of course, thoughts of failure also crept in.

The day arrived for the appointment with Dr. Spitz. After examining Doug, he said, "I don't know if what I have to offer will help, but it would be worthwhile to try." His assessment was that Doug's problems were not a genetic occurrence, as I had been told. He felt the damage had been caused by anoxia—the result of lack of oxygen at the time of the first hernia surgery.

He continued, "Doug was very little at that time, and he lost too much blood before the transfusion was administered. That caused a lack of oxygen to the brain and resulted in brain damage."

Now my mind was getting excited along with my heart, and I started to set aside all negative thoughts. I began to think maybe this was the reason we were moved to the Philadelphia area—to find this doctor. Did the Lord have a plan? Were our prayers going to be answered? Arrangements were made for Doug to be admitted to Broad Street Hospital in downtown Philadelphia for neurological testing.

During Doug's hospital stay, the nurses caring for Doug told Dr. Spitz that Doug seemed different from most of the children for whom they cared with similar conditions. One said, "He is more responsive.

There just seems to be something locked-up in there, and if we could find a way to unlock it, it might help to make a better life for him."

Dr. Spitz said he had had the same observation.

At that first examination, when Dr. Spitz had said he didn't know if what he had to recommend would work, he was referring to a program offered at The Institutes for Human Potential in Chestnut Hill, Pennsylvania. He said he worked closely with the Institutes, and many of his patients had experienced great results.

We were very excited and hopeful, and could not wait to hear about the program. We hoped and prayed that he and the nurses were correct in thinking there might be something there to unlock and that this would be the way to get to it. This was what we had been hoping and praying for since we were first given the news of Doug's severe and profound brain damage.

The program Dr. Spitz recommended at the Institutes for Human Potential is called "patterning," a process of manually moving parts of the body in a crawling motion, hoping that the uninjured brain cells will learn, take over, and help train the damaged cells. The staff reported that some patients progressed well with patterning, and there could be hope for Doug.

By this time Douglas was around six years old, and both Dr. Spitz and the Institutes said that patterning worked best for people who had already had the experience of crawling, walking, and other functions of a person with normal abilities, but who had experienced a trauma situation, such as an auto accident, which caused brain damage. Dr. Spitz and The Institutes said it would have been better to have started the patterning with Doug at a much earlier age. However, the staff and doctor thought there seemed to be something there. They said we should give it a try since we had nothing to lose.

Wrong! After starting the patterning program, I soon found there were two things I did lose: time and energy. The patterning procedure consisted of placing Doug face down on a padded table with one person manipulating his head in a right-to-left motion while four other people maneuvered each leg and arm. It was a timed ten-minute rhythmic motion with the head being the leader and the right arm and left leg moving together and left arm and right leg moving together. The movement resembled a baby's crawl.

Doug had never been through the experience of crawling. This was a new experience for his body, and he strongly objected to the activity. The Institutes recommended the use of a prod similar to what is used on cattle, gently touching his feet, one at a time, as we tried to get him to move. We objected at first, feeling it was a cruel thing to do, but the crawling was not happening the way it should. We were assured that the prod would not cause pain or harm; it would just give him the urge to push with his feet and start the crawling motion to get away from the strange sensation it gave. We were told that crawling is a very important part of learning the motions of walking and how the brain functions during the body's very early development.

Doug definitely did not like the prod, but it did get him moving. Fortunately, we did not have to use it for very long because he eventually realized that when I touched his foot with my hand, he had to push against it and keep going until I stopped urging him to push. When he wouldn't move he would get a strange sensation given by the prod.

Chapter 9

The next two-and-a-half years of our lives were pretty hectic. The patterning program also included crawling sessions, tactile stimulation, light stimulation, visual stimulation, and masked breathing exercises. While we were in the Philadelphia area, we started the program with volunteers from our church helping. Later, we were transferred back to Toledo. There we had a team of one hundred volunteers coming to our home each week to help with the patterning and crawling exercises—and lots and lots of coffee and conversation.

The patterning was done eight times a day. Doug and I started our daily routine at eight a.m., and we were busy with some part of the program until eight p.m., seven days a week. Finding the hundred volunteers and setting up the scheduling for the patterning was quite a chore. We were fortunate that a lady who became one of our first volunteers offered to take on that responsibility. She did the advertising to garner the help of family, friends, church members, and people from the community and she also helped with the patterning.

We were now settled back in Toledo and very involved with patterning. We had to take Doug to Philadelphia every two weeks for Dr. Spitz and the Institutes to check his progress, monitor his development, and add or change parts of the program. I remember those trips with my "special child" by myself on an airplane and in a taxi. With Doug not able to walk, I had to carry him, the diaper bag, and enough food, etc., to last at least a day.

At that time, there were no baby seats with handles, as mothers have today, and on some of these trips Doug would be in my arms for the whole day, from seven a.m. until evening, usually around nine p.m., when I arrived back in Toledo. One helpful side to this situation was that Doug was small for his age and weighed much less than a normal six-year-old.

I did have help on some of the trips. Sun Oil set up business trips for Cowan to correlate with the doctor visits whenever possible so he could go along and help.

The airline personnel soon knew Doug and me by name. They would see us coming through the terminal and by the time we arrived at the check-in desk we would already be checked in. The flight attendants were helpful and understanding. On many occasions when Doug was fussy, and it seemed I had done all I could do to keep him from annoying the other passengers, a flight attendant would ask if she could walk up and down the aisle with him. That worked for a while until she had her duties to attend to. Then it was my turn again.

There were times when the first-class section of the flight was not full, and we would be moved there. The seats were roomier and made it much easier to handle Doug. I could use the seat next to me as a bed for him. What a relief it was for my back and arms to be able to lay him down, even if it was only an hour or two.

The trips to Philadelphia, the doctor, and the Institutes put a great strain on our finances. We felt the Lord had answered our prayers and led us to the doctor who might be able to help Douglas, and we were grateful. We did, however, tell the Lord we really needed His help with the financial situation. We did not know how much longer we could afford to continue. On the other hand, we knew we had to continue for as long as we could financially do so, or until we got an indication from the Lord that we should stop.

Chapter 10

On the lighter side, there were fun times in our home, even during all the commotion that was taking place. Lisa started begging for a dog. We realized her life was far from other kids' typical family life. But I was not thrilled with the dog idea. Didn't we have enough to deal with and clean up without adding more? I did finally decide that a dog might be good for her and would give her some companionship. I insisted, however, that it must be a dog that did not shed.

Cowan was attending his Navy Reserve meeting one evening when one of the men in his company said his mama poodle had just had a litter of puppies. He offered one of them to Lisa. He said Lisa could have the pick of the litter. Of course, she was very excited as she looked them all over. She fell in love with the runt of the litter and said that was the one she wanted. Even though the owner tried to show her the other puppies' good qualities, she wanted that one.

Soon Fifi joined our family. They say dogs are smart. Well, this one definitely was. She knew whom she had to butter up to gain favor.

Whenever I was sitting, which was not very often, she would sit at my feet and stare up at me with a look that said, "Aren't I just the cutest puppy you have ever seen?" Yes, she did finally win my heart too. She was a delight to the whole family; except, maybe, to Doug.

I'm including Fifi's story because she gave us all a lot of joy, fun, and laughter, and because of the way she related to Doug. Lisa dearly loved her, but Doug's response to her was another matter altogether. Fifi liked to sit with Doug in Cowan's rocker/recliner.

Doug never liked to touch fuzzy or furry things, such as stuffed animals. The tactile part of the patterning was intended to acquaint him with the feel of different materials, and make him comfortable with them. At this point, though, it had not worked, and that meant furry Fifi was a no-no. The dog would jump up in the chair beside him and Doug would push her out, and back up she would jump. After the dog's many tries, Doug would breathe a big sigh, give in, and let her stay. However, Doug did not really give up and ignore her, he would start sifting through her fur and get two or three hairs between his fingers and pull them out. We watched this activity many times, and were amazed that the dog never bit him. She would just jerk her head and look up at Doug as if to ask, "Why did you do that?" Then she would lay her head back down.

Cowan was teaching a young adult Sunday school class. We decided to take the day off from patterning and invited the class to our home for an open house on a Sunday afternoon. The house and the food were ready to receive our guests, and just before the guests arrived, I put a dish of chocolate-covered cherries on the coffee table. As usual, Douglas and Fifi were sitting in Cowan's rocker/recliner. We were busily hustling around, making sure all was ready and making a last-minute tour of the house.

You've probably guessed what I am going to tell you. We found Fifi and Doug covered in gooey candy. Fifi had been getting a chocolate cherry candy and jumping up beside Doug, and then repeating the action, until there was only one left on the dish. We discovered this just before the doorbell rang when our first guest arrived. What a mess to clean up: chocolate, cherries, sticky cherry syrup, messy clothes, messy chair, messy Doug, and messy dog. All we could do was laugh and clean it up! Of course, Doug didn't eat any of the candy, and he had no clue what a commotion Fifi had caused. A few hours later, we knew for sure that Fifi had eaten it!

Chapter 11

The patterning sessions seemed to be beneficial for Lisa too. The volunteers came for the first session and stayed for the next session, which began a half-hour later four times a day. Between the patterning sessions, I would take Doug through the crawling motion on the floor to reinforce what we had just finished on the table. At that time, the volunteers would give attention to Lisa, playing games and reading to her. Part of Doug's patterning program included flash cards with letters of the alphabet, numbers, and words, which were to be recited to him in the hope they would stimulate his brain and strengthen his eyes.

The helpers would make up games for Lisa using these cards. With this attention, Lisa was reading pretty well before she started kindergarten. They would also take her to the park or for walks, and sometimes to their home for visits. These experiences gave her the ability to relate very well with adults.

There were no children close by for Lisa to play with, and my schedule made it impossible for me to taxi her around. This did not seem to bother her, though. She became good friends with our next-door neighbors, the Ardusers, an elderly couple who spent a lot of time with her. Mr. Arduser was eighty-five and confined to a wheelchair. He thought Lisa was the greatest thing since sliced bread because she loved to visit and carry on conversations with him. One day he said to me, "She really loves to talk, but that's okay, because I do too."

He taught her to play a game called African Pooh, which I still do not understand. They would spend hours playing the game and talking together. Mrs. Arduser said she did not know which one of them liked to talk the most: her husband or Lisa.

I said to Mrs. Arduser, "I think she is making up for Doug not being able to speak."

We had never heard a word from Doug, and frankly it was comforting to hear Lisa talk and be able to carry on an intelligent conversation; so the fact that she loved to talk was refreshing to me.

Chapter 12

As we watched Lisa's development with joy and excitement, we began to discuss bringing another child into our family. She seemed to be so "normal" and such a bright child that we thought maybe it would be safe to have another child.

I did have some hesitations, though. *Maybe we should not tempt fate and be happy with our family the way it is*, I thought. I spent a great deal of time again discussing Doug's situation with my obstetrician as I had before Lisa was born, and the same concerns about having another child. As he had done when we discussed the feasibility of having Lisa, he reassured us that there should be no worry regarding a genetic problem.

I prayed for resolution to the perplexing and anxious moments I felt while trying to make this decision—a decision that could have a significant impact on my life, and on the lives of my family. A quieting of my heart finally came and gave me peace in the knowledge that God was still in control, and maybe the fact that Lisa's development showed such promise was a message from Him that all would go well. We gave the decision of another child to the Lord and went about our daily activities.

Soon it was evident there was going to be an addition to our family. My obstetrician monitored me very closely during the pregnancy, determined to prevent problems. However, even before this baby was born, difficulties developed. The discovery was made that the baby was an Rh factor baby. On August 3, 1967, about three weeks before my due date, the doctor decided to induce labor and take the baby from my womb's hostile environment.

Amy, our third bundle of joy, joined our family. I was told that I had a baby girl. That pleased me, but as I waited for her to be placed in my arms, I began to fear there was a problem. She was not given to me to hold immediately as Doug and Lisa had been. As I continued to wait, I was told her birth weight was five pounds. She was jaundiced and needed a blood transfusion. I asked to see my baby and was told that I would have to wait until the transfusion was completed.

I felt a cold chill come over me and tears started to fall down my cheeks. "No, please, please not again, Lord," I prayed. The fact that I could not even see her brought unpleasant thoughts to my mind.

The transfusion was about two-thirds of the way through, and problems developed that prevented it from being continued.

As I lay there in the labor recovery room, exhausted, confused, and sobbing, I remember praying, "Lord, if you will only spare her life, You can have her to use, however, You please." How noble and self-righteous I must have felt! I remembered how Hannah in the Bible story I had heard in my childhood Sunday school days said something similar to God, and look what happened to her son, Samuel. He became a great leader for the Lord!

Amy's situation was monitored for several hours while the medical team waited to restart the transfusion. Eventually, her body started to produce its own good blood, so the transfusion was no longer needed. The fact that the Lord spared her life and that her body started producing its own good blood, eliminating the need for a transfusion, gave me hope that everything would be okay.

The nurse finally came in with my little bundle of joy—and she was a "little" one. At five pounds, she was a much smaller bundle of joy than either Doug or Lisa had been when they were given to me to hold the first time. I remembered how tiny Doug seemed, but Amy was so tiny it frightened me. She could almost fit into the palm of my hand. She had even tinier fingers and toes than her brother and sister. As I had done with Lisa, I did a thorough examination and found that everything appeared to be okay, but I did feel intimidated by her tiny size.

The custom at our church was for newborn babies to be dedicated to the Lord. Remembering what I had promised the Lord in my prayer in the labor recovery room, we dedicated Amy with thanksgiving for her life being spared. Dedication of children is for parents to promise to raise the child in a Christian home, teaching them about Jesus and His love for them. It is a commitment to be a Christian example for the child to follow. For me, the dedication was also an act of turning her over to God for his use, as I had promised.

Amy came home to join our family and all the confusion of the ongoing patterning work with Doug. Although she was very fragile, and had such a difficult start in life, she seemed to be doing well as we enjoyed watching her follow Lisa's pattern of development.

However, after a couple of months it became apparent, at least to me, that all was not well. I thought I could see a difference in her behavior. She had been holding her head up and following lights and people as they moved around the room. Now I noticed that these actions had stopped, and she was also having difficulty holding up her head. Since Amy had such a difficult start in life, I had spent my days since her birth being in watch mode, and my antennae were sensitive to this change. Something was wrong! There was a problem!

My concern became so haunting that I made an appointment with Dr. Baehren to check her. He said he couldn't see any problems and asked what made me think there was. I told him what I had noticed, but he still did not think I should be too concerned. He said she had been through such a difficult start that it was too soon to tell.

I asked if it would be okay with him for us to get a neurosurgeon's opinion. He referred us to one locally. When I called for an appointment, I was told it would be four months. No, no, that was not going to work. I wanted an appointment right then. I wanted to know as soon as possible if there was a problem. I had seen so many brain damage conditions with all kinds of tragic results on my trips to Philadelphia with Doug that I felt slightly educated on what a problem might look like.

I was going to be making the trip to Philadelphia with Douglas for a visit with Dr. Spitz anyway, so I asked Dr. Baehren if he had any objection to my taking Amy also. He replied, "No, I have no objection, but again, I don't think you will find there is a problem. You will just be wasting your time."

So Amy went with Doug and me to Philadelphia to see Dr. Spitz on the next trip, and since Amy was going, Cowan went along also. Dr. Spitz asked the same question Dr. Baehren had asked: "What makes you think there is a problem?" I told him my concerns, and after examining her he said he thought I might be right.

"Let's admit her to the hospital and do neurological testing," he said.

I felt déja vu at hearing Dr. Spitz say "neurological testing." I'd been there before, and it gave me chills to hear those words again. He suspected a tumor, hydrocephalus, or toxemia, and the testing would give answers.

"I think we may have caught this soon enough that you will not have another situation like Doug's. Let's see what the tests say," he said.

I was informed that Amy's stay in Broad Street Hospital was going to be three to four weeks. I was invited by friends from the church we had attended when Cowan had worked in Philadelphia, to make their home my home as long as Amy was in the hospital. Cowan was not with me for the testing and hospital stay. He felt he needed to save time off from work to be used to deal with whatever the results of the tests might bring.

I remember the Sunday morning in church before the testing was to start on Monday. The pastor explained Amy's situation to the congregation and asked for prayer for us during the following week. He also included her in the morning congregational prayer. I was so filled with joy at the fact that I knew the Lord was in control and would watch over her that I began to cry, and the crying continued through most of the service.

At lunch that afternoon, Evelyn said she felt so sorry for me in church, and she knew it must be difficult, but to trust the Lord. Oh, she just didn't understand that those tears were tears of joy, not tears of fear or anxiety. I was putting my trust in the Lord.

I remember one of the songs we sang that day:

How Firm a Foundation

Fear not, I am with thee, O be not dismayed,
For I am thy God and will still give thee aid;
I'll strengthen thee and help thee, and cause thee to stand
Upheld by My gracious, omnipotent hand.

When through fiery trials thy pathways shall lie,
My grace, all sufficient, shall be thy supply;
The flame shall not harm thee; I only design
Thy dross to consume and thy gold to refine.

The soul that on Jesus has leaned for repose,
I will not, I will not desert to his foes;
That soul, though all hell should endeavor to shake,
I will never, no never, no never forsake.

—John Keith, 1787

The prayer and the song's comforting words gave me God's calm assurance that He would be with both of us, and all would go well through the next days. It also backed up the quiet voice I had heard earlier, reminding me of the Bible verses I had memorized in my childhood that said God would never leave me or forsake me, and that would include Amy also.

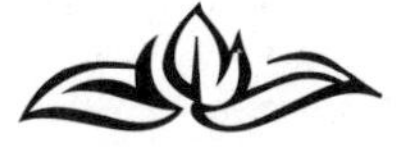

Chapter 13

The series of tests that were performed on Amy included blood tests, electroencephalogram, brain biopsies, and x-rays. The first test performed, and the one that would give the fastest results showed fluid on the brain—normal pressure hydrocephalus. The doctor explained that hydrocephalus (also known as "water on the brain") was causing an abnormal increase in the amount of cerebrospinal fluid in the cranial cavity, accompanied by enlarging of the cerebral ventricles, which was causing pressure on the brain, and could cause atrophy of the brain.

Dr. Spitz said Amy should have a V-J (ventricle-jugular) shunt put in place to reduce the pressure. He explained that more tests might uncover other situations that were causing the problem, but the shunt would need to be done under any circumstances, so it should be done while waiting for the results of the other tests. I knew nothing about the shunt. He told me it was newer procedure and explained how it worked. He said it should help by reducing the fluid buildup, which would reduce the pressure.

Dr. Spitz told me about the shunt's history. Several years earlier one of his patients had had the hydrocephalus situation, and Dr. Spitz told her parents he knew what should be done to alleviate the pressure, but there was no mechanism at that time to do it. This patient's father asked what the doctor needed, and Dr. Spitz said basically a relief valve. It so happened that the patient's father was a valve engineer and said he could design the shunt. He did, and his daughter was the first patient in whom Dr. Spitz implanted the shunt. It was successful in eliminating the excess fluid and relieving the pressure on the child's brain.

We agreed to Amy having the V-J shunt implanted. The procedure inserted a tube in the ventricle cavity of the brain and ran it alongside the jugular vein in the neck and down into the belly where the fluid drained and dissipated. A small pump was placed behind the ear that had to be pumped twice a day to keep it running properly.

This procedure continued for three years, at which time the shunt had done its job and was no longer needed. But the decision was made to leave the shunt in place rather than put Amy through another surgery to remove it. Dr. Spitz said there would be no problem leaving it in, and if, at some later time, she needed it again, the surgery would not be as extensive.

Another part of the testing was a brain biopsy. This was accomplished by drilling holes in the skull on each side of her forehead at the hairline and taking a small amount of brain tissue to be sent to a laboratory for diagnosis to address the possibility of a toxemia problem. The tissue was sent to a special laboratory out of state, and getting the results from these tests usually took several weeks. For that reason, Dr. Spitz wanted to do the shunt while waiting. He felt it was not toxemia, but wanted all concerns to be addressed. A few weeks later the brain biopsy tests report came back negative, which relieved the doctor because he said that dealing with toxemia would be very difficult.

The day arrived for Cowan and me to hear the explanation of all the test results. I was beginning to feel like an expert at waiting for and hearing test results. As we arrived at the doctor's office, I felt a little tense at what the tests would have to tell us. I searched Dr. Spitz's face to get an indication of what I was about to hear. I was anxiously looking for a smile, a satisfied countenance, or something to let me know everything was okay. But, what I saw was a concerned, expressionless countenance. This caused me to take a deep breath and stiffen my body—which I was also becoming an expert at doing—to get prepared for what he had to tell us.

The results: brain damage. The diagnosis for Amy, the same as Doug's, severely and profoundly brain damaged—retarded."

I was not ready for this news again. I felt my mind racing and my heart pounding just as it had when we were given the good and exciting news that Dr. Spitz might have help for Doug with the patterning, but this time it was not excitement that brought the racing and pounding, it was hurt and disbelief. *Could this really be happening again? The same diagnosis!*

I will never forget the scene when Dr. Spitz gave us the news. A nurse was sitting very closely beside me, which I thought was strange at the time, but what I did not know was she was holding smelling salts out of concern about what my response might be. Maybe they could see my racing mind and hear my pounding heart so I suppose they expected me to pass out from the news. I don't know why, but that did not happen.

As Cowan and I entered the elevator to leave, I said to him, "If this is God's will," which I knew it was, "I pray that in some way He will receive honor and glory from it." God had to be giving me strength because thinking back on that day; I do not understand why I was not a basket case at hearing this news again.

Again, the news went out across the miles to family and friends: "We have another one of 'heaven's very special children.' Amy has also been diagnosed as severely and profoundly brain damaged. Please pray with us that we will be able to take on this responsibility, and do it well."

A cloud of frustration and confusion hung heavily over me as I prayed, "Lord, I promised you could have her to use, but severely and profoundly brain damaged? How can you use a brain-damaged person?" You would think that having been through a similar situation with Doug, I would have been used to receiving this kind of news, but it hurt just as much as the first time. One was a trial, but two brain-damaged and helpless children? *I don't know if I can do it*, I thought.

I tried to deal with the news, another Bible verse, Philippians 4:13, made its way to my memory: "I can do all things through Christ who strengthens me." I knew this was God answering the "how can I?" question in my prayer. I was now beginning to understand the importance of, and to be grateful for, the memorizing and hiding of those Bible verses in my heart.

I had thought in my early years that Bible memorization was a useless effort. Now I realized that those verses certainly are helpful and comforting at very important and distressing times in life. I know that all things that happen in our lives have a purpose. Testing and trials are to grow our faith. Bible verses were helping make my faith stronger.

I began to understand that sorrowing for what had happened was looking backward. There was no need to dwell on it. I could not change it. Worry for what was yet unknown meant looking around. There was no need to be searching and concerned for what might be. I could do nothing about it, even if it came. Faith looks up, and there I will find all I need to have my concerns cared for, and my hurting heart soothed.

I now had to accept the fact that I had two helpless children, and also Lisa. I was still certain that the Lord had a plan for all our lives. So we needed to get on with the patterning, and the changing and feeding of two helpless ones, and make life as normal as possible for Lisa.

Accomplishing these tasks in addition to cooking, cleaning, and other mother and homemaker duties presented overwhelming and exhausting challenges on some days. But God was gracious in giving me the strength to meet the challenges. On the day Amy was to be released from the hospital, Dr. Spitz's intuitions must have told him that our thoughts were probably going back to being told that Doug's situation was genetic because he reassured us again that the circumstances with Doug and Amy were not genetic— especially since Lisa was very normal. The conditions were unrelated.

He also said, "You will continue to be told by doctors that it is, but doctors are human and can be wrong."

I asked him if we could do patterning with Amy as we were doing with Doug, and he said, "No, she is much too fragile." He added, "We probably should consider stopping the patterning with Doug."

We discussed that we were not getting the results we had hoped for. He asked what I would consider to be a success if we were to continue, and I told him that if Doug could just walk it would be a great help.

"That might be possible," he replied, "but it might take another ten to fifteen years of patterning to get to that point, and then we would have to be concerned about him getting into dangerous situations, such as touching a hot stove, etc., because he would not have the understanding that there was danger."

He was also concerned about what effect patterning had had on Doug, and how having another child so severely involved at the same time would affect the family. He said, "You have done what you could to make a difference for Doug. You can always know that you did all you could. If you had not done the patterning, later in life you might think you should have at least tried, but you can be sure of the fact that you did something."

Cowan and I spent a lot of time praying and discussing the pros and cons of continuing the patterning, and the concerns Dr. Spitz had discussed. We decided it was probably time to stop. I have no regrets for the two-and-a-half years of travel, the financial burdens, the hours spent in doctor's offices, and the time spent patterning, because we truly felt it was what we were being led to do at the time.

There was one positive result of patterning for Doug, though. The masked breathing exercises made his respiratory system much stronger, and the bouts with respiratory infections dropped significantly. We were thankful that at least patterning had improved his health.

Chapter 14

The confusion and frustration I felt caused my mind to start asking questions. But these questions that were trying to work their way into my mind seemed to be different from the "little quiet voices" I had heard so many times before that brought Bible verses I had memorized to mind. Those voices gave me encouragement, but these were giving feelings of discouragement and defeat.

Why the discouragement? I wondered. I realized it was Satan trying to put in his two cents worth by planting these questions to weaken and destroy the faith I had been holding onto. One of his favorite thoughts to use was, "Maybe you have not been good Christians." I also realized that Satan was the reason for my questioning God whether I could carry on with the responsibilities of two special children.

"You cannot continue with two children with so many needs. It will be too difficult for you," Satan whispered.

I made a determined effort to resist and block those thoughts, saying, "Satan, move away. Leave me alone. I can do this. Why not us? We are trying with God's help to be the Christian parents He expects us to be, and since God is in control here and He has said that we can do all things, with His help I know I can do it."

A battle between encouragement and discouragement was taking place. At the same time that Satan was trying to put discouraging thoughts in my mind, I heard a quiet voice that I had heard many times say, "Don't you know all things work together for good to them that love the Lord and to those who are called according to His purpose?" as it says in Romans 8:28.

"But, Two, Lord? Can I really do it?" I asked. Satan was trying to discourage me so I would give up.

But then the reassuring, quiet voice said again, "It's for your own good."

Wait now, how can it be good for me? Satan was trying to make me see, just like that teacup in the antique shop, how my life was bogged down with such a load that it might be my destruction. But the Lord kept coming back with "for your own good, for your own good," which was puzzling to me.

The battle going on in my mind between Satan and the Lord continued to come and go. However, the Lord did win the battles.

I know now, and I actually knew then, that if I had given in to Satan's temptation and let him be the ruler of my heart and mind by listening to him and responding to what he wanted, the consequences for my children and me would have been a disastrous journey. Instead, it has been a journey of victory that has given me a sense of worth.

While I was trying to deal with "for your own good," again the small voice whispered, "Not only for your own good, but what about the rest of the verse: 'to those called according to His purpose'?"

"Yes, I know that is also part of the verse, but, how this will be good for me," I responded.

I was trying to understand these "conversations" with God when finally I had to say, "Okay, Lord, if it is for my good, which I cannot see now, I will trust you for that good. But there is a purpose too?"

I knew Jesus told us that whatever we ask for in His name, He will give—if it is within His will and for His purpose.

"But, Lord, I ask you to help me understand," I said.

It was time again, actually the third time, for the doctors to bring up the subject of institution, now not only for Doug but for Amy too—"because you cannot manage two completely helpless children, and remember, you have Lisa to worry about," they said. It was true that Doug and Amy were helpless and their care was intensive and time consuming, and we too were concerned about how this situation would affect Lisa, but our answer again was, "No, institutionalization is not the answer. God has a plan for their lives and we will let Him help us work it out. He will have to be the one to show us if and when that decision should be made."

I mentioned earlier that well-meaning people started to ask a lot of questions at one point, and this was that time. "How do you feel toward God because of these trials?" they would ask. My answer was then, and has always been, "God did not cause this to happen. However, He did allow it, and there must be a reason."

I am sure their comments were meant to show compassion for what—in their perception—was an unbearable situation for us. We appreciated their genuine concern. We tried not to give a reason for others to have feelings of sympathy for us. That was not what we wanted.

The next test of faith came when sympathetic people would confront me to ask, "How can this happen to good Christians like you? Aren't you bitter toward God for allowing this to happen?"

Since I was blocking Satan from using my mind to plant these thoughts, it seemed he was now using others to do it for him.

"Bitter?" I asked. "No, I am not bitter. What has happened is either to prove our faith in God, or a process of drawing us closer to Him."

I have since found that it was both. Even when conditions as devastating as these "trials" came into my life, I could still have faith and trust in God's all-knowing will, and heaven knows it drew me closer to Him. I had to lean heavily on Him for the strength I needed to get through each day.

CHAPTER 15

There was usually chitchat around the table during the ten-minute patterning sessions. One day while we were at the patterning table, there didn't seem to be much chitchat going on. Trying to break the silence, one of the ladies managing Doug's left foot said she could not understand why conditions such as these happen. Another lady said, as she nodded her head toward me, "I know why she is going through all this."

What? I thought. You better believe my ears perked up, and I listened and listened well since she was clearly going to share some insight I had not quite received. She proceeded to tell us she had been having difficult times, and during some of those times she thought she could not go on, but then she would remember me and what was happening at my house. She continued, "I finally decided if Janice can do all she does with these special children and Lisa, and still have a good outlook and exhibit such faith, I can also get through what I am faced with."

Without realizing what I was saying, the words came out of my mouth, "Thank You, Lord, if this is the way you are using me and our family." Wow! I was shocked at what I had just said: Thank You, Lord, for using us to help others through their tough times! That thought had never crossed my mind, but if the Lord was using our two special children, and the two-and-a-half years of patterning, to help others in some way as they dealt with situations that came into their lives, I would give Him praise and thank Him for helping us to be useful. I was now beginning to see and feel bundles of joy that were coming from my bundles of joy.

During one of our trips to Philadelphia for a follow-up, Dr. Spitz noticed that the electroencephalogram showed Amy was starting to have seizures. I had watched her have some trembling, but since it had not resembled Doug's violent actions when he was having the seizure on that snowy morning many years earlier, I didn't think about it being seizures. Her actions were quieter and with less movement, the most obvious when her eyes rolled back.

A medication treatment was prescribed to keep the seizures under control. After treatments for the seizures had been going on for about six months, we again started to feel the financial crunch of doctor bills and airplane fares. Also, we were not seeing much change in the seizures or progress in Amy's development and began to question. We had asked the Lord for guidance in the matter and felt we were supposed to be seeking this help for Amy. Now we were praying for specific evidence that we should continue.

At the very next visit to Philadelphia, the electroencephalogram showed that the seizure activity was much improved.

"We thank and praise you, Lord," we prayed. "You have answered our prayers, and the seizures are improved, but please show us some way to deal with the financial situation."

On another day as we were patterning and having our usual chitchat, I was asked if we had ever thought of contacting the March of Dimes for financial help. No, I had never thought of that as an option, but I was willing to pursue any avenue of help available. I called the March of Dimes and gave my story. They asked me how much we would need for the next trip to Philadelphia. I provided the details, and to my surprise I was told there would be a check in the mail that day to cover the expenses for the next trip. The gentleman on the phone said he would present our situation to their board of directors for further consideration.

You cannot imagine how far off the floor my feet were walking for the rest of that day! Two days later the check arrived, and he called back and told me the board of directors had met and discussed the circumstances we were facing, and their decision was to pay the plane fare for as long as they could financially do so.

What joy! The Lord had graciously answered our prayer. We were very grateful for the help we received, and to show our appreciation we have contributed to the annual March of Dimes fund drive almost every year since. For the past several years I have helped the fund drive by being a neighborhood captain, mailing fund-drive request letters, and receiving the donations to be sent back. My desire is that God will use our contribution, and those of the neighbors to whom my letters are mailed, to help other families in their time of need, as He did for our family.

During my visits to Dr. Spitz, I witnessed brain-damaged people ranging from infants to grown-ups. I would look around the waiting room, which I had plenty of time to do because we were usually there for a three- to four-hour wait at each visit before we were called into the doctor's office, and I would see circumstances I felt were worse than mine, and that would have been much more difficult for me to handle. When our turn came for Doug's examination, I mentioned this to Dr. Spitz, and he said, "You are right in that feeling. If all my patients' problems were put into a bag and shook up, each parent would reach in and take back their own."

Looking around at all the different scenarios, I thought to myself, *yes, he is right.* My situation was heartbreaking, time-consuming, and exhausting, but seeing what other parents were dealing with made me grateful for my situation. Some of these patients were higher functioning, walking around and keeping their parents busy trying to keep their child out of trouble. Some had temper tantrums. Some made loud noises over which they had no control.

My thoughts went back to the time when Dr. Spitz said, "You don't want Doug walking around if he doesn't understand danger and how not to become involved in it." I knew how exhausted I had been at the end of some days, and my heart went out to these parents who had to manage these hyperactive children, in addition to the kids' mental disabilities, and most of them were patterning their children also.

Describing to our friends the situations I would observe at these doctor appointments prompted me to say, "I would rather have my two children in their condition than have them be borderline and higher functioning." There was always shock and disbelief when I made the comment. The comments would be along the line of, "You can't mean you would rather have such totally disabled children, rather than have them be able to have some capabilities."

I continued to say it also made me feel glad to know that they never would realize that people were staring at them or laughing and making fun of them, and feel the hurt that can cause. I have seen hurt, embarrassment, and humiliation in the eyes of borderline "special children" who do have some understanding of their circumstances when others laugh, stare, or make fun of them. I have also seen the deep hurt their parents show. I could feel the stab in my heart that the parents were feeling in their hearts as I watched the hurt look on their faces.

I'm not saying those stares did not happen with Doug and Amy, but they never were aware of it, and even though at times I felt a stinging hurt myself, I just told myself that the person did not understand. I can truly say I have never felt embarrassment or humiliation for the appearance or actions of my bundles of joy. They are not mistakes at the hands of God. They are His creations—jewels to love and treasure.

Chapter 16

Douglas and Amy came into the world at the time when "special children" were just beginning to be taken out of hiding, so to speak. The norm had been to shelter them in institutions, as we had been advised to do, usually in a rural area far away from society. I mentioned earlier that my children went with the family to Sunday school and church every Sunday, but they also went many other places, such as to the park. They traveled with us to many more cities, not just to their doctors in Philadelphia, and they shopped at the supermarket and mall, and visited friends. They even went "out" with us on New Year's Eve.

Our family and four other families rotated homes celebrating New Year's Eve every year. Doug and Amy were always included in these celebrations. Doug loved loud noises, so you can imagine his delight at the noisy celebrating on New Year's Eve. Even though they were not able to participate in the activities, they seemed to enjoy just being there and hearing the fun and excitement their mom and dad were having. They certainly were not sheltered, nor were they intentionally put on display. They were just our kids.

I said, they went food shopping with me, and that was a sight to see; Doug sitting down in the shopping cart and Amy in her baby seat perched in the child seat area of the cart. Since Doug was not fond of touching things or having things touch him, keeping items in the shopping cart was a challenge. I don't remember eggs ever hitting the floor, but I became a pretty good "fly ball" catcher of all kinds of items. I caught them most of the time!

Doug, Amy, and I made our weekly shopping trip to the supermarket. They were sitting happily in the shopping cart as I was trying to find places to put items where Doug could not pick them up and throw them. I heard a commotion in the next aisle between a mother and child that did not sound happy. Apparently, the child wanted something, and the mother said no. The child screamed and cried, and Mom would either ignore him or tell him no again, usually in a loud, angry voice. At one point, I think she must have slapped him, which she had already said she would do if he did not "shut up." The child's cry changed from a begging cry to the cry of hurt.

When I had completed my shopping and was in the checkout line, I realized the person in line in front of me was the mother and child who had been causing the commotion I had heard. I'm sure you know what is at the checkout point at the supermarket: candy! Of course, the child wanted some, and again his mother said no. The child continued to beg and cry until she slapped him across the face and told him to "stop acting so stupid." This time I knew for sure it was a slap because I saw and heard it.

I had had it! Listening to the confrontations all through the store, and now knowing for sure of the slap, I said to her, "You should be happy he can speak his mind and be responsive to you. You are very fortunate." She turned and at first glance gave me a glaring look as if to say, "What business is this of yours?" When she was fully turned around, probably to have some choice words with me, or to ask me to mind my own business, astonishment came to her face that turned to embarrassment when her eyes fell on Doug and Amy. Having some difficulty in not knowing how to respond to my comment, she finally said, "I don't know what to say except I am sorry that you have this situation to deal with, and I am ashamed of my actions."

I continued through checkout and found she was waiting for me outside. She apologized again. She seemed genuinely interested and asked about the problem with my children.

I told her, "Nothing! They are perfect for our family, and have brought our family much joy."

I did proceed to tell her the diagnosis and the fact that they would never talk, walk, or feed themselves. They were blind and not toilet trainable.

She turned to her little guy, gave him a hug, and told him she was sorry for being so mean to him. Then she turned back to me and asked, "How do you do this all this by yourself?"

I told her I did not, that my husband and I have Someone who gives us all we need to be able to love and care for these bundles of joy.

She said, "You must mean God, right?" to which I replied, "Yes, every day and night."

She thanked me for being able to discuss my "trials," as she called them, with her. She said, "You have been an inspiration to me, and I know you will be to others."

My hope is that she has been able to be more patient with circumstances in her life, and be thankful for her "normal" child. Maybe my "special children" were part of the education for this mother and also for others to help them become acquainted with and understand people who are mentally challenged and retarded. This incident and the discussion at the patterning table (the lady who said she felt she could get through troubling times in her life when she remembered what was happening at my house) caused me to wonder if God could be using our family to help others. I asked for guidance and understanding as I began to search the Bible to find answers. Three passages came to my attention:

> He helps us in all our troubles, so that we are able to help others who have all kinds of troubles, using the same help that we have received from God.
>
> —2 Corinthians 1:4 GNT

> Consider yourselves fortunate when all kinds of trials come your way, for you know that when your faith succeeds in facing such trials, the result is the ability to endure.
>
> —James 1:2-3 GNT

> Do not be surprised at the painful test you are suffering, as though something unusual were happening to you. Rather be glad that you are sharing Christ's sufferings, so that you may be full of joy when his glory is revealed.
>
> —1 Peter 4:12 GNT

These verses took my thoughts back to that day in the elevator after Dr. Spitz had given us the news that Amy's tests showed severe and profound mental retardation, and I asked the Lord to use Amy's situation to bring honor and glory to Him. Was it possible that in my effort's praise, honor, and glory were being given to God? When situations presented themselves for which I needed to ask Him for strength and help, I felt humble, and at the same time filled with joy. He was using our family to reveal His love and grace.

I had many more similar "conversations" with the Lord. I suppose I was getting to the place where the teacup was when it said to its master, "Stop it. Stop it. I'm burning up. I'm being patted and patted. I'm spinning round and round," and the teacup's master only shook his head and said, "No, not now."

Even though I never audibly said, "Stop it, stop it," my thoughts probably sent the "stop it" message to the Lord. At times, I certainly did feel like I was on a potter's wheel with my mind spinning round and round as a result of the incidents that continued to occur.

Many times during those days I found myself asking for strength and help. At other times, when I could feel God's arms holding and comforting me, I gave thanks for His loving care.

As I read and reread these verses and had "conversations" with the Lord, I said, "Whatever is your will in this, Lord, I will accept it and again ask you to show me how to use our events to bring honor and glory to you through it." Then that quiet voice I had heard many times before returned to say, "I will never leave or forsake you, and remember you will never be given a burden too great for you to carry. I will be there with you." My prayer became that I would be like the teacup—a finished product useful to the Master for whatever purpose was His will.

People asked how the situation with Doug and Amy affected Lisa, and if we felt sorry for her. When I turned the control of our lives over to the Lord, Lisa was definitely part of that trust. It was not easy for her to have her mother away in Philadelphia so often, and having so many people in and out of our home with all the activity that went with the patterning. We tried to be as truthful as we could with a five-year-old child. We explained to her, in a way she could understand, that the situation with Doug and Amy was not a sickness that could be treated with medications, and that would someday go away. This was the way it would probably be for the rest of their lives.

Chapter 17

In 1970 Cowan came home from work with the news that Sun Oil was transferring him back to Philadelphia, and this time we knew it was to be a permanent move. We had enjoyed the previous year-and-a-half assignment and the friendships we had made in Philadelphia, and we looked forward to the move.

The company made plans for us to fly to Philly to start our search for a home. We had dedicated four days to the house search. From the list of houses that had been sent to us for review, there was one house in particular that interested us, but the real estate agent did not want to show it to us. She said, "That house is in such bad condition; I'm sure you would not be interested if you see it."

We finally had toured all the houses on the list we had received, except the one we had the most interest in seeing. The end of the four days of house hunting was fast approaching, and we still had no place to live. We knew we did not want to make another house-hunting trip, so we told the agent that we wanted to see the split level house that was on the list, and if she did not want to show it to us we would get another agent to do it. She finally gave in and made the appointment.

How right she was! It was in horrendous condition, but it turned out to be the house we had dreamed about—a very large, five-level home on a hill and in the woods. We purchased the house, completed the move, and the extreme makeover began. We scrubbed, cleaned, removed wallpaper, painted, removed walls, removed and installed new flooring, and did all the other tasks that go along with moving into a house in such a state to make it our home. It was a shame that the house was in such poor condition when it was only eleven years old. We wondered how a house could get into such disrepair in such a short time.

Several months after our move back to Philadelphia, Sun Oil also transferred our very close friends Jon and Sharon Helms to Philadelphia. Jon and Sharon were our first, and only, matchmaking effort. (We stopped while we were ahead.) Jon worked with Cowan, and Sharon and I were neighbors and walked to school together. We were convinced that they were right for each other. We were best man and matron of honor at their wedding, and that matchmaking effort has lasted for fifty years.

Sun Oil put them in touch with the same real estate agent who had worked with us. As she was showing houses to them, she found out we were friends. She said to Jon and Sharon, "Your friends, the Browns, are crazy for moving into that house. It will take their whole lifetime to get it in shape."

To make a long story short, several months later we invited her to lunch at the home, and she was flabbergasted at the change. She said, "You should be a Realtor—you could see the possibilities that I did not, and being able to show those possibilities to buyers goes a long way toward helping a Realtor become a success."

Little did she or I know at that time that years later I would become a real estate agent.

One of my assignments after getting the family settled in our Philadelphia home was to get our phone service set up. A young man, probably in his early twenties, arrived to do the installation. I noticed he made several trips up and down the stairs to each phone, and he would always come back to the phone in the kitchen, which was next to the living room.

As usual, Doug and Amy were happily lying on the floor in the living room. It seemed to me that the young man should have been finished with the set up much sooner, but the trips up and down continued.

Eventually, on one of his trips to the kitchen and living room door, he asked if he could ask a question. "Of course," I said, and he asked,

"What is the problem with your children? I notice they stay in one place and are not very active."

I told him their diagnosis and asked why he was asking.

He proceeded to say that he and his wife had only been married a short time, and they had been discussing whether or not they should have children.

I asked him why what he saw of my children would have anything to do with whether or not they should have children.

They were seeing so much evil in the world, he said, and so many terrible incidents happening all around us, and now he saw our situation. "Our discussion has been if we should bring children into the world to face all these things. We know it will only continue and get even worse," he explained.

My first thought was that this couple must be responsible young people, which I'm sure they were.

I said to him, "I understand your thoughts, but let me leave two thoughts for you and your wife to consider. First, life can become very lonely with no family to enjoy it with, especially when you get to your senior years.

Secondly, even though the situation you see here with my children may seem tragic, if you never have children, you will never feel the joy of holding a little person that you know is a part of you. To you it may seem like an insurmountable task to care for these children, but I would not want to have missed it."

I asked him if he was a Christian, and he said, "Yes, and we go to church."

"Then you must know that God has told us that He will never allow us to carry a burden alone," I told him, "He will walk through it with us. He has helped me through my circumstances, and He will deal with all the evil that you and your wife have been discussing."

He thanked me and said I had given him something for him and his wife to think about. I have wondered many times what their decision about having a family turned out to be.

Our move back to Philadelphia was in June, and it soon became time to enroll Lisa in first grade. I wanted to give her as much attention as I could to show her that she was just as important to me as Doug and Amy—so I volunteered to be homeroom mother. I was responsible for setting up parties and other activities for special occasions.

At the Halloween party, the teacher and I were talking as the kids enjoyed their treats. I felt the need to tell her about Lisa's home situation, thinking that might help her to have a better understanding of Lisa. She said she already knew about our special family, and that Lisa was the one who told her. She proceeded to tell me that, during the first days of the school year, her policy was to ask the children to tell about their families—how many sisters and brothers were in their family, what their father did at work, etc.

She noticed Lisa did not have her hand up to be first to speak, and that was unusual. Finally, she asked Lisa if she wanted to tell the class about her family. She said Lisa came to the front of the class, planted her feet firmly on the floor, gave a big sigh, looked the children in the eyes, and said, "Yes, I will tell you about my family. I have a brother and a sister. They cannot play with me or argue and fight with me and all the other things you say your brothers and sisters do, because they are brain damaged. They will never be able to walk or talk. They cannot take care of themselves or play with me, but I love them anyway."

Her teacher said Lisa gave the description of her family to the class with an inflection in her voice, and an attitude of, "And you better be okay with that." She asked Lisa if she would like to tell the class what it meant to be brain damaged—and Lisa gave a beautiful explanation.

The teacher told me I did not have to worry about Lisa's understanding and acceptance, because she certainly understood. She said she looked around the room while the Lisa was talking and the students sat mesmerized. There were many tears, including her own.

Another activity, the first-grade teacher practiced each year was to have each child tell how old their parents were, and what they did at work. At the first Parent-Teacher meeting, she said to Cowan, "I have been waiting to meet the 103-year-old father of a six-year-old child in my class."

On the day after the assignment was given, Lisa had asked Cowan how old he was. Cowan asked, "Why do you wanted to know? I am

103 years old." So when Lisa gave her family report, she told the class her father was 103 years old!

Lisa gave us much joy and pride as we watched her grow and saw what she could accomplish that was impossible for Doug and Amy. She was the part of our lives that helped keep sanity in our home. She was a delightful child to raise, never giving us grief or concern. Cowan and I have discussed many times that she probably was such a great child because she realized we had a pretty full plate with Doug and Amy, and she didn't want to add to that burden. There were never complaints about the situation at home and the fact that our family could not do the things her friends' families did. We have said many times that God gave her to us as a consolation prize.

Lisa was a great board game player, even at a very early age. One of her favorite games was where one player pulled pegs on their side of the game piece, trying to make the discs, they cannot see, hanging on that peg of the opponent's side fall off the peg. She and her dad played the game day after day and she would always beat him. He kept saying he could not understand how she was able to beat him every game they played. Not sometimes, but always! She would just smile and enjoy the victories.

One day, however, I guess she felt sorry for Dad, and she said, "Dad, do you know how I beat you all the time? I can see the discs on your side in your reflecting in your glasses, so I know which peg to pull." That was the end of Cowan wearing his glasses when he played that game with her, and he did win some games after that.

Chapter 18

In 1972, we received a letter from the state with information that was a total surprise, and that we never dreamed could happen. The letter gave us notification that the Intermediate Unit would be starting an education program for the mentally challenged, and Doug and Amy were to be enrolled in the program. *What? A school program for Doug and Amy! You have got to be kidding me!* We finally came back down to earth, but were still excited that this could be a possibility. *How can that be? What can they learn?*

The program was mandatory, so soon our children were off every day on the school bus to "school." Knowing that parents would be confused and curious, the Intermediate Unit invited us to watch a demonstration of what the "schooling" would be. It showed how our children would be involved in activities such as hand-over-hand dressing (a staff member would take the hands of the students and move them to perform), brushing teeth, brushing hair, playing musical instruments, doing artwork, etc.

I have already mentioned that I had doubts that Doug and Amy were at a mental level where they could "learn," but we certainly were willing to give it a try. Anyway, we did not have a choice in the matter, because it was mandatory. With the children off to school every week day, I didn't know what to do with myself. Not having the chores of feeding, changing, and keeping them occupied, I completed my household chores by ten a.m., and I found myself with nothing to do.

The freedom was great, and the opportunity to visit or go to lunch with friends, go shopping by myself, or work in the yard helped to take up some of the time, but soon those activities did not totally satisfy. I began to think about going to work, but I had not worked since I was in college unless you count the years of raising three children—two of which were "special children"—as work.

Instead, I decided to find volunteer work in the community. Two volunteer opportunities were recommended for me to consider, and they both sounded very interesting. Several ladies from my church were volunteering on the women's auxiliary board at Eastern Baptist Theological Seminary and Eastern College, and asked if I would join them. That sounded like a worthwhile volunteer activity that would occupy some of my time.

The auxiliary's main function was to provide assistance to the seminary and promote the seminary to churches in the Philadelphia area. These tasks were accomplished by inviting ladies from area churches to luncheons at the seminary, which we prepared and served. These luncheons were followed by meetings in the chapel with music, usually presented by students, and a guest speaker.

The ladies from my church, most of whom had helped me many times with the children, of course, knew my story. At one of our monthly meetings they would tell the other board members about my family. The board asked many questions and seemed genuinely interested in the activities involving my children. Their interest in my family led to my being asked to be the speaker at one of the luncheons.

Be a speaker? I didn't think I could do that. However, after some objecting, and at the insistence and encouragement from the board, I agreed. That experience went well and wasn't as frightening as I anticipated. As a result, I was asked to give the same message at several of the ladies' churches who attended that day. The ladies on the auxiliary board and other ladies from the churches who had attended said they would like to know more about my children and other experiences I had with them. They urged me to write a book and tell more of my story. The thought would cross my mind now and then, but I resisted.

The second volunteer opportunity came when a friend at church, who was a social worker, approached Cowan and me and asked if either of us would be interested in volunteering to be on the board of directors to help start a new Christian agency for the mentally retarded. She said the State of Pennsylvania had issued a judicial mandate to close the state's mental institutions and place the residents in community living arrangements (CLAs), also called "group homes." She and other Christian social workers felt the need to set up a Christian agency for residents coming out of the institutions. After all, as Christians, we should be the first to step up to give help to those who had a need—to be God's helping hands here on earth.

Since I now had time on my hands, Cowan thought I should be the one. I was to be the "user representative," representing my children and others with mental disabilities, and their families. This would be a new experience for me, but I felt it would be a good way to give back to the system that was helping Doug and Amy. I spent some time with the others who were considering becoming board members, praying for guidance and discussing each of our concerns. We all agreed that this is what we should do, and I felt it was the right volunteering situation for me at that time.

The CLA/Group Home concept was new, at least to me. The idea was to provide housing in neighborhood homes, which were to be run as if the residents were living at home with their families. There would be house parents and three to five residents. Part of the design was to teach the family members, who had been just existing in the institutions, how to care for themselves, function as part of a family, help around the home, and, hopefully, be able to participate eventually in some way in the community. What a great idea! Giving back to the community!

We started our monthly meetings, and the first item on the agenda was to select a name for the agency. The name we chose was Association of Concerned Christians for Emerging Social Services, to be known as ACCESS. Our next duty was to write a proposal to submit to the state, outlining our intentions. The next few meetings were interesting. We were given a blank piece of paper to start writing the proposal. We looked around the table at each other and saw blank faces. Where do we begin? Part of the proposal was to present a budget. Of course, we realized that this project was going to require money, so that blank piece of paper showing a zero balance became the faith part of the project. Finally, after about four months of monthly meetings, we were ready to send our proposal to the state. It was accepted and we were ready to go!

Most of the social workers on the board had been to the institutions as part of their jobs. I decided that if I was going to be helping set up homes for these people, I should go see for myself what their living circumstances had been. I was shocked; they were living far away from society, behind locked doors, with bars on their windows and living in rooms with rows and rows of beds. All of them looked forlorn as they stared blankly into space. I was told many of them never had visitors, not even family members. And this is what the doctors wanted for Doug and Amy! I don't think so!

My heart was heavy as I drove home and dealt with the thoughts that kept going through my mind. *They do not deserve this kind of life. They deserve friendship and love and to be able to enjoy the beauty of God's creation. That cannot be done behind closed doors.*

At that point, I knew ACCESS was doing what God would want us to do. The process of dispersing individuals to homes started, and as we waited for our charges, we began to search for suitable housing to rent for our homes. That proved to be a difficult and discouraging task. Most "neighbors" did not want, as they called them, "those people" living in their community next door to them and their children.

I was asked me to represent the Board at a hearing involving a property ACCESS was considering to rent. I was appalled by the questions I was asked and the cold and callous attitudes toward human beings just because of mental challenges over which they had no control, and that were certainly no fault of their own. What the neighbors would not listen to or even try to understand was that "those people" were much more frightened of living next door to them, the neighbors, than the other way around. For years before this mandate was issued, "those people" had been secluded away from society behind closed doors. This change was going to be a very traumatic and frightening experience for them.

I sat through the hearing thinking, *is the dream of being God's helping hands for His "special children" becoming a nightmare for ACCESS, and more importantly for our prospective residents?* What a shame and disgrace that they were not welcomed and shown the respect and care they deserved. Why wouldn't the neighbors understand that their children or grandchildren could be one of "those people" at some time in the future? How sad and hurt it made me feel that "those people" the neighbors did not want to accept could be my children—Doug and Amy.

After we secured homes and moved our residents in, the next function for ACCESS was to make routine visits and monitor the care and progress of our "families." As I watched the homes develop and watched our residents, most of whom exhibited abilities that were not being developed in the institutions, I thanked God for giving me the opportunity to be part of ACCESS. We watched people who could not make eye contact, could not dress themselves, and could not begin to do a chore blossom into worthwhile people who were very proud of themselves and what they could accomplish. Many times I thought, *if their families could see them now, they would be so proud.* The board felt pride in what we observed, and we were satisfied that we were doing a good job for the Lord and for those who we took as our responsibility.

By the end of the first year, starting from that blank piece of paper with a zero balance, we were proud to report to the state that we had six homes in three counties, all doing very well, and we presented a budget of $1,000,000 for the following year. We were quick to give the praise to God, because without His help and guidance we could not have accomplished so much in such a short time. I am thankful that because of Doug and Amy, I was able to be part of making a better life for heaven's other very special children.

I became involved in another volunteer opportunity as an outgrowth of the association with ACCESS—participating in a caring and sharing group. The group was formed for parents who had been through similar situations of caring for their mentally disadvantaged and retarded children to help parents of newly diagnosed children cope with their circumstances. I learned about many different feelings those parents had, which were foreign to me: anger, guilt, *why me*, pointing the finger at the other person ("what did you do to cause this?"; "what did I do?"); "I don't understand and really do not want to cope with this"; and anger with God for causing the situation. My heart ached for these parents because I knew what they were going through. I remembered how difficult it was for me to deal with the kind of news they had just been given. I saw marriages and families breakup because they could not cope with the situation. Divorces happened because one or the other parent could not take the pressure and left.

While seeing these responses, I also watched families who stood up to the task and did a fine job. Part of my function was to counsel these brokenhearted families, telling them I understood because I too had been through the pain they were feeling. We felt very blessed that the Lord had guided us through our times of trial and disillusion, and had given us what we needed to deal with these trials so we could get through them without negative emotions. God is an awesome God, and I do not know how one can face events such as these and navigate through them without His help.

I enjoyed the volunteer work, but Cowan thought I should do something that gave me compensation for the time and effort I had been giving to volunteer work. While studying at the University of Toledo, I had worked at the local real estate board, giving assistance to the agents in their daily business activities. I could see the satisfaction of the agents when they were able to bring sellers and buyers together and take a transaction to a successful closing.

I have always loved to meet new people and thought this might be a way to do that. Our close friends Bruce and Mary Lou Hudson owned a real estate business and mentioned that they were so busy that they could use help. I happened to mention my time spent at the real estate board office, and how much I enjoyed it. I said that I had thought about becoming a Realtor. That comment brought this comment; if I would get my real estate license I could work with them. I went to school, got my license, and became involved in listing and selling houses. I quickly understood why the agents with whom I had worked years before found it to be so satisfying. Watching happy and excited faces on closing day certainly does give pride and satisfaction.

Chapter 19

I was very fortunate that my health was good while dealing with Doug and Amy's conditions. However, two health issues did haunt me over the years. The first was back problems from slipped discs, which I was told was most likely a result of lifting and carrying the children. I would have two or three bouts a year that took me off my feet and put me in bed for two weeks at a time, some of those times in traction.

These occasions presented the question: How do I care for Doug and Amy? We were fortunate to have friends—ladies from church and neighbors—who jumped in to help by meeting the school bus, bringing them in, and getting them settled until Cowan came home from work. Bringing Doug and Amy into the house was a challenge. Our house was located on "that hill" we had dreamed about, and that put the house thirty feet up from street level, with a long, steep driveway to negotiate.

The school bus could not negotiate the hill, so the volunteers would meet the bus at the bottom of the driveway, put them in their car, drive up to the house, bring them into the house, change their diapers, etc.

These angels of mercy would also either bring our dinner or prepare it while they were there. We were truly blessed to have dedicated friends who helped in this way. I am very much aware that God placed our family where we needed to be because He knew there would be special people in the suburbs of Philadelphia, who would be His ambassadors.

My second health issue was a dislocated shoulder. One day as I was riding a bicycle, I lost my balance, sending the bike and me tumbling over and over until I ended up on the ground in a lot of pain. A trip to the hospital emergency room revealed a dislocated shoulder. Cowan had just had spinal laminectomy and back fusion surgery and was not allowed to drive or ride in the car, so we called on our neighbor to take me to the hospital. While the doctor was working with me to put the shoulder back in place, the admitting nurse handed the paperwork to my neighbor to fill out.

Of course, he didn't have information to give them and told the nurse he was not my husband. There were some strange looks from the staff at this disclosure.

That bike "ride" was the beginning of many more dislocated shoulder incidents. The second shoulder incident happened at church during choir practice. I fell down three steps coming out of the choir loft. I knew immediately that I had to go to the emergency room, and now! Again, Cowan was not available. He was out of town on a business trip that time, so another male choir member drove me to the hospital. We went through the same scenario as the first time—no husband to fill out the paperwork. Eyebrows were raised and questioning looks were displayed at being told, the second time, that this man was not my husband.

The third incident occurred when Lisa and I were taking tennis lessons. The doctor had neglected to tell me that I should not be playing tennis, golfing, swimming, or bowling because that kind of activity might cause the shoulder to dislocate again, and the tennis did it! I was returning a backhand serve and as my arm dropped limply to my side, I felt my shoulder dislocate. Lisa looked at me over the net and knew immediately what had happened. She was not driving yet, and Cowan was again out of town on a business trip, so another tennis student (male) drove me to the hospital.

This time Lisa was with me. When the nurse started with the paperwork scenario, and jokingly said, "I suppose this is not your husband either," Lisa spoke up and said, "No. He is a friend, I am her daughter, and everything is okay."

The nurse said, "She does have a husband though, doesn't she?" And that caused all of us to have a good laugh.

During this third incident, the orthopedic surgeon told me the next time I ended up in the emergency room with the dislocation, he would have to operate. The description of what he had in mind was not something I wanted to go through. I was told that the tendon that crosses the shoulder and holds the joint in place had been stretched so many times it had lost its elasticity. It would have to be brought back over the shoulder joint and stapled to the bone. Ouch! I would then be in an airplane cast for about ten weeks. Upon hearing that, I told him he would never see me again! How would I manage Doug and Amy?

Many years went by before the next trip to the emergency room. When I arrived at the emergency room that time, and saw the doctor coming into the room, the first words out of my mouth were, "Forget it, you are not going to operate."

After putting the shoulder back in place, he said I must have learned how to live more carefully with so many years passing since the last incident. No surgery was required at that time. The thought of going through surgery made me very aware that I did have to learn how to function using the arm in a different manner, and to this day I am still very careful as to how I use my arm.

These incidents caused havoc around our house with Doug and Amy's care, especially dressing and changing diapers. I was back to needing help with school bus time. Each time the shoulder dislocated, my arm was put in a sling attached to my body. Even though it was the right shoulder, and I am right handed, I could do a fair job of feeding them with my left hand, but that was about all. Dressing and moving them was out of the question.

My shoulder became a constant aggravation, dislocating a total of eight times. It dislocated several times when I was by myself. I'd had enough experience with the situation by then to know that I had about fifteen minutes to get to the emergency room before I would get lightheaded on my way to passing out. The pain could get pretty excruciating.

With that thought in mind, I knew I did not have time to call someone and wait for a ride or an ambulance so I would drive myself. I had to steer with my left hand, and all the while my right arm would slowly move up and across my chest, ending up wrapping around my neck. Even though I tried, I had no control over it. The arm just did its own thing!

The nurse who met me at the emergency room entrance was shaking her head in disbelief. She said, "The next time you try that you are going to choke yourself before you get here."

We both stood in the doorway laughing at how ridiculous I looked. It appeared as if I was trying to hug myself. Soon she noticed that I was starting to get wobbly and she knew what that meant, so she quickly put me in a wheelchair and whisked me off for the tugging session to put my arm back in place. A tugging session was truly what happened.

The way my dislocations happened were different from what others said happened when their arms would dislocate. For me, the bone always went inward to the breast. My friend who had several dislocations told me her bone would protrude outward. She could usually put it back in herself by rubbing her shoulder gently against the wall and allowing it to pop back. That did not work with my dislocation.

The process for putting it back in place was for the nurse to roll a sheet into a tube and put it under my armpit, stand behind me while I was lying on the table, and tug with both hands on the ends of the sheet tube while the doctor took my hand and forearm and pulled in the opposite direction. By this time, I was at the point where I would watch the room go round and round and the pain would make me go in and out of consciousness. It was interesting, though, how the pain would instantly be gone as soon as I felt the bone pop back in place, which would sometimes take about ten minutes of tugging.

Chapter 20

Amy's life presented many anxious times for our family. I remember getting in the car with her one rainy day. Her leg bumped against the column between the front and rear doors while I was trying to get her into the car quickly. She made a little whimper, but then everything seemed all right. She slept well that night, but in the morning I noticed the leg was reddish and a little swollen. I took her to the emergency room, where X-rays showed the leg was broken.

The leg was put in a cast, and when time came for the cast to be removed, I mentioned to the doctor that I was apprehensive about handling her. He told me not to worry about that—a bone never breaks in the same place twice. He said the break area would be the strongest place in her body.

Sometime later she was lying on the living room floor and I heard a crack as she turned over. It sounded to me like a bone cracking. I took her back to the emergency room and tried to explain that this happened as she was turning herself over. Sure enough, when X-rays were taken, her leg was broken in the same place.

The hospital staff started questioning me as though they thought she had been abused. What a horrible feeling after the care we had given her for anyone to think we would abuse her! Fortunately, her pediatrician was in the hospital, and was summoned to check on her situation. I told him how I was being questioned. He told the hospital staff that he could vouch for the fact that abuse was totally out of the question. Since Amy was so fragile, and doctors feared there might be more broken bones, they decided to do a whole body skeletal study. To my and the doctors' astonishment, they found bones many other places in her body that had broken and healed that we did not know about.

Another one of our anxious times with Amy was when she was released from the hospital after getting through a bout of pneumonia. I was told pneumonia was a concern for a child so fragile who weighed only twelve pounds at the age of twelve.

These comments made me very nervous and, again, cautious while handling her. I became more and more concerned as she did not seem to be recovering very quickly. The main problem we faced was feeding time. It was getting more and more difficult to feed her. She would cough and choke, and it would take an inordinate amount of time to finish a meal. It got to the point that I dreaded her breakfast, lunch, and dinner times. I could see that she was getting weaker and weaker, but I attributed it to the pneumonia, thinking it had sapped a lot of her strengths.

I became concerned that she might be coming down with pneumonia again. One day as I was feeding her, the choking became so severe that I called the pediatrician, described what was happening, and asked him what to do. He told me to bring her to his office immediately so he could check her. When we arrived, and after a quick check, he said, "I am calling an ambulance to take her to Children's Hospital. She is in bad shape."

I called Cowan, who was at work in Philadelphia. I followed the ambulance in my car, and when we arrived at the hospital, Cowan and Pastor Hutchison were waiting for us. I was glad to have them there because I could tell by the doctor's response as she was being taken out of the ambulance that the situation was probably not good.

The emergency room doctor started to do his assessment, and after asking us many questions, he realized Amy was probably being overmedicated with seizure medicine. The reason she was choking and having difficulty swallowing was that her systems were shutting down. She was not able to swallow. She was dying.

A doctor from Russia was giving a seminar to interns and doctors at the hospital on overmedication and its effects. The seminar was presenting newly discovered information regarding seizures. Knowing that Amy's condition seemed to be exactly what the seminar was covering, the emergency room doctor asked the Russian doctor to assess her and give his opinion.

After his examination, he said, "Yes, this is what I have been teaching in my class."

The doctor called the whole class into the room and said, "What you see here is a classic example of what we have been discussing—overmedication and its results."

Fortunately, he also had been discussing the remedy for the condition. He directed the nursing staff to stop all medication until further observation was completed. He asked us about the history of her seizures, and then told us and the class that Dr. Spitz was doing what he should be, to control the seizures at that time and that he should not be blamed for this situation. A new medication program would remedy the situation.

What had been happening was that each time the seizures worsened, the medication to keep them under control had to be increased. The situation had been having a snowball rolling downhill effect—going round and round, and getting bigger and bigger until it crashed. The seizure medication had to be increased time and again, until Amy's body "crashed", and she has ended up here, and in this condition.

In the short time between the emergency room examination and her admission to the hospital, Amy started going downhill fast. IV's were started to give her body nourishment, and we were told they did not know how long she would live. She was in a coma.

I prayed, "Lord, I have tried my best to take care of her, but now I place her in your hands."

Cowan and I went home and started discussing her final arrangements. We went to the hospital day after day and saw no improvement in her condition. It was difficult to stand by and see no signs of life.

Amy was just our lifeless child, hooked up to all kinds of needles and monitors. It reminded me of the situation when Doug was in the hospital after his first hernia surgery at five weeks of age when he was unresponsive and I was waiting for him to wake.

One day during our visit, while standing at the foot of Amy's bed, the doctor told us that since she had been in a coma so long, they would only leave the IVs going for one more day, and if she did not respond by the next day, they would remove them.

We went home and poured out our hearts in prayer and sent prayer requests to family and friends. If she was not going to be getting nourishment through the IVs, and she could not eat herself, what was going to happen?

Reluctantly, and fearing what we might find, we returned to the hospital the next day. The nurse met us as we exited the elevator. She told us the doctor wanted to see us as soon as we arrived. My heart sank, and a big lump came in my throat. *Is this it? Have we lost her?*

As we entered the doctor's office, we were met with a big smile, and he said he had good news. And good news it was! He said, "Amy must have heard what I said to you yesterday, because she woke up this morning and has eaten a little food, and the IVs have been removed—at least for the time being."

Apparently the IV nourishment had given her body time to start healing, and she was now able to swallow. I had heard that the last bodily function to shut down when a person is near death is hearing. Maybe the doctor was right—maybe the swallowing and her body's other functions seemed to have already shut down, but she had heard his comments. However, I chose to think it was the prayers of many prayer warriors for God's intervention that brought her to "life" again.

The doctor said, "From a medical standpoint, she should be gone, but it just wasn't her time. There must be something for her to do."

My mind traveled back to the day she was born, when she was in danger, and I told the Lord He could have her to use however He needed if He would just spare her life. *Yes, He must still have something for her to do!*

Amy's recovery continued to go well from that point, and it was finally time to take her home. She was still very frail and fragile. A new prescription plan was ordered for one-quarter of the medicine that had caused her near-death situation. This medication was newly on the market for seizures and was not available in pill form. It had to be formulated as an elixir.

During a check of hospital discharge instructions, someone discovered that the prescription was written incorrectly. Instead of being written for one-fourth of the original, it was written for double what it should have been. Needless to say, there were some anxious doctors and staff! We all breathed a sigh of relief and were thankful it was discovered before we took the prescription to the pharmacy.

We arrived home, and Cowan took the prescription to the corner pharmacy. With his chemical engineering background coming into play, and before giving Amy the medicine, he read the directions, did some calculations, and realized it had been filled incorrectly. Instead of being filled for one-fourth of the medication that had caused the problem, it had been filled for four times the amount of the hospital's prescription.

He took the medicine back to the pharmacy, and when the pharmacist looked at the label on the bottle and again at the prescription, Cowan said he turned as white as a sheet and said he was glad we had not given her the medicine. It would have killed her instantly, he said. Here again, as the doctor said after she came out of the coma, it just wasn't her time.

Friends asked us if we would still be using that pharmacy. The answer was yes, definitely. We were pretty sure that the pharmacist would give special attention to us when we brought him a prescription after that incident.

Chapter 21

Speaking about medications, I sure do appreciate applesauce! Doug and Amy have both been on medications most of their lives. The only way we could get their pills down was to bury them in applesauce, which, fortunately, they both liked very much. However, there was a period of time when we had to watch Doug closely at pill time. He would swallow the applesauce and spit out the pill.

How strange that he knew how to do this! How did he figure it out? It would have been a blessing if his ability to distinguish between applesauce and pills and how to separate the two could have been present in other areas of his life.

Doug and Amy had kept the doctors, hospitals, and pharmacy very busy for many years when another family member joined them in these activities. In 1979, Cowan developed chronic cluster headaches and spent the next fifteen years in agony. He took heavy medications to try to get relief from the pain. The medications would lessen the pain somewhat but would never completely take it away. Doctors told him that the cluster headaches are one step past migraines in the pain they cause, and they are the most difficult to find a treatment that gives relief.

The fact that the cluster headaches were chronic gave him very little time free from pain. He sought the help of many doctors, clinics, medication programs, acupressure, and acupuncture, but found no true relief. The pain was so intense that he was willing to try any suggestion given to him just to find some relief.

The medications were pretty heavy hitters, and would often put him into a zombie-like state for days at a time.

One day Lisa came running to me and said, "Something is wrong with Dad. He is sleeping, but he is laughing and mumbling."

She and I were both concerned as we watched what was happening. I called the doctor and he told me not to give any more of the medication, and he wanted to see Cowan the next day. It was determined that Cowan's system could not tolerate Valium, one of the medicines he had been given for pain.

On another occasion, Cowan asked me what the date was. I told him, and he said, "That is scary. The last day I remember is —" and the date he told me was the day two weeks earlier. That was not only scary for him; it was frightening for me, as well.

Unfortunately, this was not an isolated occurrence. It happened frequently. The headaches began to have an effect on his work. He would lose one to two weeks at a time when he could not go into the office because of the pain and/or the effects of the medications. When he would decide to try, many times he would just turn around and take the next train back home.

He began to feel he was not giving the company a full job for the salary he received, and that worried him a great deal. Doctors had told him that stress might be part of the cause for the headaches. He finally decided if his concern was causing stress, and if stress was causing the headaches, quitting work was one thing he could do to control it.

He explained his concerns to his boss. The boss and the company were willing to work with him to keep him on the job, saying that at forty-three years old, he was too young to retire. However, his concerns became so worrisome that he and the company mutually decided that disability retirement was best.

Chapter 22

I mentioned earlier that there were lighter times in our complicated and confusing household. An activity that caused laughter was when Lisa found that if she opened an encyclopedia, held it close to Doug's ear, and slammed it closed, causing a loud thudding sound, he would go into such laughter that it caused everyone in the room to laugh along with him.

When Lisa saw his reaction, she could not stop with just one slam. The first slam would be a surprise to Doug, and cause him to jump at the sound, laugh, and then cock his head and ear in the direction of the sound and wait for another slam, laugh again, and wait again. Most books would make a sound, but the encyclopedia, being such a large book, made the loudest sound, and produced the biggest laugh. It reminded me of his swinging on the front porch when he was a toddler and the neighborhood children making him laugh by pounding on the porch floor.

Amy liked sounds also. However, quieter sounds were her speed. If Lisa approached her ear and whispered, "Amy Beth Brown," she would go into hilarious laughter. Once she composed herself, she would do as Doug, tilt her head and ear toward Lisa with a mischievous grin and a gleam in her eyes as if to say, "I'm waiting for another 'Amy Beth Brown.'"

Lisa said, "Watching that mischievous grin and the gleam in Amy's eye; I think that if she were normal, I would have a little imp for a sister."

Amy was our noisemaker. Lisa would complain about times of aggravation with Amy, when she would be watching a TV program that was of interest to her, and Amy would make her noises, usually not stopping until the commercials came on. Amy was more active and "mouthy" than Douglas, and her "talking" consisted of outbursts of loud noises. She would make noises at inopportune times. It was interesting how the dog responded to her. Fifi was never quite sure about Amy and what she might do, so the dog would ignore her and walk all the way around to the other side of the room to get past her.

I have been asked how many diapers I thought I had changed over the years with my children. That would be very interesting to know. I had at least one in diapers for twenty years, two in diapers for thirteen of those twenty years, and during some of those twenty years there were three.

In the beginning days of my diaper changing, they were cloth that had to be washed and dried. I had to wash and rinse them several times with each wash to be sure the soap was gone so the kids' bottoms wouldn't get red and raw. Eventually, even the duplicate washing and rinsing did not work, and the doctor told me I would have to start using disposable diapers.

I balked at that idea, mainly because of the cost. He told me I really had no choice if I wanted healthy bottoms for Doug and Amy. He gave me a letter of prescription for disposables, and told me to save the letter and all the store receipts for the disposable diapers and claim them on our income tax as a medical expense.

I was not sure I really believed that could be done, but I filed the letter of prescription and started buying the disposables, saving the receipts in the file with the letter. At tax time, I had to put the doctor's suggestion to the test.

Cowan's debilitating headaches made it impossible for him to concentrate well enough to do our taxes, so I did them myself that year. I was a little apprehensive about claiming the diapers as a medical expense, but I had done as the doctor said and saved the letter and receipts. I included them in the tax return.

Yes, we were tagged for an audit. I took the letter of prescription and the store receipts and arrived at the IRS office at the appointed time. The lady doing the interview said, "Do you know why you have been called in for this audit?"

I said, "Well, I'm not sure, but is it because we claimed disposable diapers as a medical expense?"

She replied, "You are exactly right. You cannot claim them as a medical expense."

Since I was pretty certain the reason we were being audited was because of the diapers, I had gone prepared. I had used the tax handbook to prepare our taxes and found that the doctor was correct. I brought it with me for proof that I was legal. I told her to look at a certain page and section, and she would see that I could claim prescribed diapers as a medical expense.

She opened to the page and section and to her amazement she found that my claim was legitimate.

She said, "You are right. I did not know this to be so." Then she added, "However, while I have you here, let me ask you about your giving. No one gives this kind of money to the church."

I came prepared for that too. When I took the canceled checks out of a shoebox and showed her we did indeed give that amount to the church, her mouth fell open. She was speechless. She finally said, "You may go," Actually she said in a kind of joking way, "Go on. Get out of here." She could probably tell from the shoebox full of canceled checks that I most likely could respond to any other "you cannot do that" comments.

Several people told me I should keep very good records because what usually happens after an audit is you will be audited for the next three years. I never heard from the IRS again—yet! It pays to be prepared! And, no, I still do not know how many diapers I changed, but it seemed like multi-millions.

Chapter 23

Lisa was a tremendous help to me when she reached an age where she could feed and change Doug and Amy and sit with them as I ran errands. I think these experiences helped prepare her for a career in nursing. She is now an ICU nurse.

She has always been a very good diagnostician in medical situations. She suffered for many years with bouts of fainting from terrible abdominal pain. It seemed it always happened when we were at the dinner table. She would instantly pass out and fall to the floor. We consulted many doctors, and thinking she probably had an allergy, they performed extensive rounds of allergy testing to two hundred items—but no allergies were revealed.

One day, Lisa came excitedly into the kitchen where I was working and said, "I know what my problem is and why I am passing out."

I asked how she knew.

She replied, "The television program I am watching is discussing lactose intolerance. My passing out and the other symptoms I have been experiencing_are a result of intolerance to lactose products. I am not going to drink milk or eat cheese or ice cream any longer."

I knew she was convinced, because she loved ice cream. She did stop eating the dairy items and that was the end of the passing-out experiences. Upon checking into lactose intolerance, we found that the reason she was passing out was that when she ate a dairy product her intolerance caused the pain to become so severe that the way her body would deal with it was to pass out. Fortunately, Lactaid milk for lactose intolerance was just being introduced. She started drinking the milk, felt better, and had no more passing out situations.

When she was starting college at East Carolina in Greenville, North Carolina, we were concerned that she might not be able to find Lactaid milk there. We made contacts with all the supermarkets. None carried it. Since we could not locate Lactaid milk in the area supermarkets, we searched for other avenue. The only place we could find a Lactaid product was at a pharmacy in pill form. The pharmacist assured us that he would keep it on hand for her, and he did.

Another area where Lisa was, and still is, a good diagnostician is with automobiles. She would stand by and watch her dad work on our cars. She was also observant when noises and problems arose and would ask the why and how-do-we-fix-it questions.

While she was in college, Lisa worked at the corner market during the summers. She usually parked in front of the barbershop in the shopping center. Bob, the barber, said he would watch her come out from work and when her car wouldn't start she would get out of the car with her ponytail bobbing, open the hood, do something, get back in, and away she would go. He said he could never see what she did, but whatever it was, the car would always start.

Several times when she came home from school for holidays she would tell her dad this or that was wrong with her car. Cowan would ask how she knew that was the problem, and she would say, "It's making the same noises or actions your car did when it had that problem." They would take the car to the mechanic, and she would usually be right in her diagnosis.

One day Cowan said to her, "Honey, even if you are pretty sure what the problem is, when a guy has car trouble, never tell him what you think is wrong—and especially not on a date. Men will not appreciate a girl giving them a car diagnosis. It's a guy thing!"

Chapter 24

Cowan was returning to work from lunch one day in 1974 when he noticed a trip to Copenhagen for Sun Oil employees posted on the message board. The price was so incredibly reasonable he decided to make arrangements for us to go. He was planning to surprise me and tell me just a few days before we were to leave. But when he mentioned this great opportunity to friends, they told him he should let me know because part of a trip like this was the excitement of the planning and the anticipation.

I'm not sure he had thought about what to do with the children, but our friends also told him they would take them while we were away. What a joy and blessing to have friends who would take on such a responsibility, especially with Doug and Amy. Barbara and Earl Russell kept Amy, Suzanne and George Murr kept Douglas and Fifi, and Grace and John Harron kept Lisa. Of course, we had a wonderful trip, and we had no worries about our children—we knew they were in good hands.

Our friends said everything went well in caring for Doug and Amy (and Fifi). Lisa, however, had the trauma of her bunny, Handsome, dying, and Mom and Dad were not there to comfort her.

The Murrs told us we had a weird son and dog. There had been a terrible storm while we were away and their children and dog were terrified. Meanwhile, they found Doug sitting on the bed laughing and Fifi lying sound asleep on the floor by the bed, oblivious to the storm noise.

On another occasion we needed someone to care for the children while we were away. Other friends, Cliff and Ginnie Johnson, offered to care for Douglas. Ginnie's mother, Mrs. Collier, lived with the Johnsons, and she was fascinated with Doug, especially watching Ginnie feed him.

One day at dinnertime, Ginnie approached Doug with a plate piled high with spaghetti which was, along with applesauce, his favorite food. (Fortunately, we had passed the split pea and ham Gerber land baby food era. Thank You, Lord!) Her mother said, "You are not going to feed him all of that are you?"

Ginnie said, "You just watch."

After each bite and before he hardly had a chance to swallow, his mouth was wide open for the next bite. Ginnie's mother said, "If you keep going he will burst."

After he had eaten all of it, her comment was, "I would have never believed it."

These two incidents were not the only times these eight friends and their families were ready to step in and help whenever and wherever the need arose. Their giving spirits have left footprints on our hearts that can never be washed away. Those times of comfort and help they gave to our family bring to mind the poem "Footprints in the Sand." The poem says Jesus picks us up and carries us when our burden gets too difficult to carry alone. That was certainly what our friends did for us. They were, and still are, a blessing.

I should back up at this point and share what happened to Cowan not long before we left on the trip to Copenhagen. Going to the train to go to work, with icy conditions, he slipped, fell, and was knocked out for a few moments. When he came to, he got to his feet and continued on the train to work. He did not seem to have any immediate effects from the fall. However, the day after we arrived home from Copenhagen, he could not get out of bed due to back problems. He would spend weeks at a time on bed rest and sometimes in traction to, hopefully, put an end to the problem.

The bed rest and traction continued for several months but did not help. His orthopedic surgeon said Cowan was going to need a spinal laminectomy. Knowing about our situation with Doug and Amy, he said Cowan's back would need to be fused. If the fusion was not done, he would not be able to lift more than about five pounds, and both Doug and Amy weighed more than that. Cowan tried to wait it out, and give his body time to heal, but eventually the surgery became the only route that was going to give healing.

Cowan does not remember much of what went on during those five days after the surgery, other than getting to the point of asking for something for the pain. The drugs would then put him back into a state of limbo. The doctor told us Cowan could not go back to work for at least six months. This was not pleasant news because he had already lost three months trying to solve the back problem before having surgery. But the doctor said the jerky train ride to work could possibly undo the good that the surgery had done.

Cowan did not like the idea of being so limited, but he certainly did not want to go through surgery and physical therapy again. "Once was more than enough for me," he said. So he took the doctor's advice and spent the next six months recuperating.

Several years following Cowan's surgery, Amy started to develop scoliosis curvature of the spine. She was beginning to lean acutely to the left, very close to the arm of her wheelchair. As we watched her lean, and watched what it seemed to be doing to her body, we realized something had to be done. The doctors were concerned that if the curvature continued it would involve vital organs: liver, kidneys, and maybe even the heart, which might cause serious problems.

An evaluation suggested that a spinal surgery should be done—surgery similar to her dad's, but in addition two metal rods would need to be inserted, one along each side her spine. It was distressing for us to watch the curvature's progression, but we were very hesitant for such serious surgery to be performed. It seemed we were in a catch twenty-two situation—possible problems if we allowed the surgery, and definite problems if we did not!

Cowan said, "Absolutely not." Since he had been through back surgery and knew the pain he had experienced, he was not ready to watch Amy suffer as he had, especially if there could be any other way to remedy the situation. The doctor was persistent in telling us it must be done. But we were also persistent in our decision of no, not yet, not if there is any other way to stop the curvature.

We asked what the percentage of success would be if the surgery were performed, and how dangerous it would be. He said the surgery should be successful in correcting the curvature, but then came the down side to the surgery—there was a fifty percent chance of causing permanent paralysis, or even worse. I did not want to ask what he meant by that comment. We were definitely not ready to take those chances.

We searched other avenues for a remedy, and found evidence that full-body casting might be a viable option. Our search showed that casting had been successful to correct curvature situations for many patients without surgery. We told the doctor that we wanted to try the full-body cast before taking the route of surgery. He was not as excited about casting as we were, but finally agreed that it would be okay to try. He had doubts that it would work, and said we would be losing valuable time.

The body cast started under her arms and went down to her hips, and was hinged so it could be removed at night and for bathing. She was required to have a cast on during the day or whenever she was out of bed. It did not seem to bother her, and it did make her sit straight and tall. Actually, she looked much more comfortable. The doctors agreed to Amy continuing to wear the cast, and that they would do assessments every few months. She wore the cast for five years, having it resized as she grew.

At the five-year assessment, the doctor decided to leave it off for a time and see what would happen. We were overjoyed to see that the curvature had stabilized, and the cast would no longer be needed. The doctor was impressed and pleased with the results also. We were glad that we had not made the decision for surgery, especially with the chance of permanent paralysis—not to mention having Amy to go through the painful process of surgery.

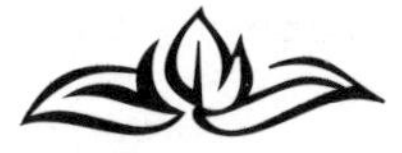

Chapter 25

In 1975, bubbles and floaters started developing in Cowan's retinas, which led to several laser surgeries. We were told that the bubbles were a precursor of hemorrhages. The laser surgeries left scarred areas in the middle of his vision.

On June 11, 1976, his right eye hemorrhaged. He called his ophthalmologist, head of the Retinal Clinic at Jefferson Hospital and Wills Eye Hospital, and gave him the news: "I can't see out of my right eye."

The doctor said, "I was afraid of this, but sharing that fear with you would have just added to the anxiety and tension, which may be part of the problem. What you are experiencing is hemorrhaging."

Normally, the doctor said, if you can get through two years of the plasma bubbles, they often subside before retinal hemorrhages.

Cowan had made it to April 1978—one year and nine months—before the retina hemorrhaged. The hemorrhage caused bilateral loss of central vision and left a ninety-five percent reduction of vision in the eye. At this point, he was declared legally blind due to macular degeneration. No more driving and he would have a lot of difficulty reading. His glasses were fitted with a telescope to help him read, but the viewing area was so small that he could read only one or two words at a time, which made reading a painstaking task, and very tiring.

An amusing side to the telescoped glasses is that Cowan gets special attention when he goes into a jewelry store. The salespeople think this man must be an expert on diamonds!

The doctors felt the bleeding was aggravated by physical and/or emotional stress. There was plenty of both of that in our home.

We were told he could no longer lift the children, as it would cause physical stress, and he could not take the emotional stress of watching me do all the lifting. I am sure that even the thought of my doing all the lifting definitely would have been stressful for him. Due to lifting them, he had watched me spend a couple of weeks two or three times a year in bed with slipped-disc back problems.

At the doctor's suggestion, he sought advice from clinics and retinal specialists throughout the northeastern part of the country, and they all agreed that the situation was permanent and blindness was probably coming. There was no cure. He was told the blindness would not get to the point that he would be walking into walls, but it would definitely cause very limited activity.

The laser treatments stopped the bleeding, but unfortunately left scarring that caused blind spots in his central vision. He enjoys telling people, "I'm not really as shifty-eyed as it may look. I just have to look at you sideways." For him to look at someone and see the face, he has to look at that person from the peripheral area of his vision. On occasion people will think he is not paying attention to them—that he is looking off into the distance at something else.

The ophthalmologist knew the situation in our home, and our intention of never placing Doug and Amy in an institution unless it became absolutely necessary because of physical, medical, or emotional problems. So the ophthalmologist told me, "Unfortunately that time has come. The children have to be removed from your home. This is definitely a medical and emotional situation. It's your husband or your children."

What a dilemma—my husband or my children! Even though we had rejected the suggestions of institutions over the years, we realized we were not in total control of events in our lives and the decision to place them outside our home might have to come someday. We just were not ready for it right then.

We had turned that decision over to the One who knew what was best for all of the family, and began to realize that this might indeed be the time of His choosing.

A friend worked at a private home for mentally retarded and challenged persons. Knowing our children might someday need the services offered there, she had told us that if and when a time like that came, she knew Doug and Amy would benefit from living at Melmark, located in Newtown Square, Pennsylvania. She had nothing but praise for the care she saw given to the residents.

We drove through the grounds and liked what we observed. We kept asking our friend questions about the facility and continued to be pleased with what we heard. She checked with the admissions office and was told the waiting list was three to five years long, and we should put Doug and Amy's names on the list if we were considering ever making Melmark their home. We told Cowan's ophthalmologist that Doug and Amy were on the waiting list at Melmark, where we wanted them to move when the time came, but the waiting list was about three to five years.

The doctor said, "No, it must be immediately, you cannot wait."

Melmark said there was a three-to-five-year waiting list, and the ophthalmologist said we could not wait for those years to pass, so I started on a mission to find a home for Doug and Amy. We knew it would have to be a special place, similar to Melmark, because we had invested too much of our lives and love into Doug and Amy's lives to let it be lost. The time-consuming activity of searching out and touring facilities showed very limited possibilities that I would even begin to consider for the care of my children's precious lives.

Just in case something might change, we made an appointment with Melmark for a tour of the entire campus and to have an interview. As we toured the campus, we could see and feel the love, care, and concern for the residents, as our friend had described it, much different from other homes I had just toured. As we watched the activities and the staff and aides, we could see the professionalism in their respective positions. The residents were happily hustling and bustling around, and at the sight of our new faces, they gave us unconditional acceptance into their space, and I even got a hug. A happy place to be sure!

I lost my heart at Melmark that day, and I knew immediately that this was the place I wanted Doug and Amy to call home.

Melmark's beautiful campus is located in the suburbs of Philadelphia. The home is a fantastic, very large French Chateau mansion with many wings and several floors with many rooms. Each time I entered the foyer of this home, I was in awe of the grand circular stairway. There was an outdoor and indoor swimming pool, horse riding ring, and many acres for expansion. By most standards, it would be labeled an institution—it is located in a country setting, but that would be the only feature that would correlate to the institutions I knew about. I can testify that it is far different from what I saw at the institutions I encountered while on the ACCESS board. It was also different from what I saw on our search for a facility for Doug and Amy.

The residents in this facility are treated like family, with aspirations for their growth, development, and happiness in life. To the staff and caregivers it is not just a job, it is a dedication. I appreciated the fact that this "job" was only done by compassionate and dedicated people.

For our interview we met with the president and CEO, Paul Krentel, who along with his wife, Mildred, were founders of Melmark. Mr. Krentel was familiar with ACCESS and the philosophy surrounding the establishment of group homes. He also had been told that I was, at that time, vice president of the ACCESS board. He asked me, "How can you want your children to live here, when you are actively involved in placing others like your children in group homes, which are very different from what most people would call Melmark—an institution. Don't you feel like a traitor?"

My response was, "First of all, Mr. Krentel, no, I do not feel like a traitor. Melmark certainly is not an institution as I know and have seen institutions to be. There is a place for every kind of situation with the retarded, and I think that Melmark can serve my children's needs the best. Since they cannot feed themselves, cannot walk, cannot talk, and are not toilet trainable, how can they function in a group home set up for the growth and development of those who are able to do these tasks? Secondly, I know how expensive group home living is, which is much more than the costs of care here would be."

I knew this to be true because setting up budgets for group homes at ACCESS was part of my job as a board member, and Cowan and I had been receiving information on the cost of living at Melmark. I was not in agreement with government money being spent unwisely, especially when there was an adequate alternative.

"And thirdly," I went on, "I want my children to have a home where there is the love and care we have witnessed here."

I am not sure he ever fully understood where I was coming from and why, but Doug and Amy were approved for Melmark to be their home. However, he informed us that there were no openings at that time. Understanding the urgency of our situation, he said he would see what could be done.

Chapter 26

It seemed as though there were situations causing anxiety at our house again and again. There had been many times of discouragement. Cowan's diagnosis as legally blind and the fact that he could no longer lift Doug and Amy was definitely a time of discouragement.

I was discussing this with Pastor Hutchison one day.

"Haven't we been through enough? Haven't we done a good job? Are we still being tested?" I asked.

His response was, "Sure, you have done a good job. In fact, you have done an excellent job. Yes, I think you have been through enough, but yes, maybe the Lord is still testing. You will never know the number of people who have been watching you as you have dealt with these trials, and to whom you have been an inspiration without you even being aware. Maybe the Lord now has something else for you to do."

Our pastor had walked with us through many hours of the trials and frustrations, but also through the times of joy, and we treasured his wise counsel. He proceeded to ask me if I would consider being the speaker on Children's Sunday and share my experiences. I asked why. He told me I needed to be telling others how the Lord has walked with me and our family through all the trying circumstances, and how He had given us the strength to do what needed to be done. Then he said, "Maybe it's time to testify of the love, comfort, and strength He has given you to help you through those rough times."

"I cannot do that," I told him. "That would be bragging, and I would never use my children as a platform to brag. Also, I would be too nervous, and I don't know if I could keep composure while talking about things that are so personal."

He said, "The one you would be bragging about is the Lord, not yourself, and I know you well enough to know that you are thankful for His presence and guidance. Don't you want to tell others? There may be others who need to hear your story to help them through difficult times in their lives." He asked me to think and pray about it and let him know.

This conversation brought back memories from two earlier times. One was of the conversation at the patterning table when the lady said she had been able to get through difficult situations when she remembered what was happening with me. The second was my confrontation with the lady and her son in the supermarket. Both of these people had said I was an inspiration to them.

Well, maybe he is right, I decided, *and I should be sharing my journey and the guidance and help the Lord has given to travel the roads of joy, love, laughter, trial, and discouragement.* As I considered his request, my thoughts drew me back to those Sunday school days and the lessons that told us to go and "tell the story" of Jesus' love. I prayed as he suggested and finally felt the Lord giving me assurance that He would be there with me.

On Children's Sunday I shared the story of my "Bundles of Joy" and the bundles of joys they had brought into our home—the same speech I gave later at the luncheon at Eastern Baptist Theological Seminary, and to several other churches as a result of my association with the seminary.

Chapter 27

We continued our search for a suitable facility for Doug and Amy that would be available immediately. However, my heart and mind were at Melmark. I toured many facilities throughout the state of Pennsylvania and came to the realization that none of the ones I had seen were, in any way, going to compare to Melmark. We knew the doctors would continue to insist that Douglas and Amy must be removed from our home, but this was not an easy decision to make, and not one to be made hastily.

After searching and touring and exhausting all options for a satisfactory home that would resemble Melmark, we chose another facility while we waited for our children's names to come to the top of the Melmark list. We had made the difficult decision of choosing a facility, but now we faced another difficult and very important question. How were we going to pay for this care?

We had been receiving pricing information from the facilities I had toured and realized we would need help. We searched for a source of funding and became discouraged because none seemed to be available. A friend who had influence in our county started helping us with the search, and suggested an avenue he felt might work.

We applied and waited and waited, but nothing happened there either. Our friend recommended that I hand-deliver a handwritten letter to the possible source of funding, explaining in detail our family and the circumstances we were facing, and let the Lord use the letter to bring financial help. He and I both thought that a personal, face-to-face contact might get a more positive response.

When I delivered the letter, I was asked to give a brief synopsis of our situation. A couple days later a phone call came, saying we were approved for the monthly charges to be paid. We felt God had answered our prayers, and that this confirmed the move for Doug and Amy.

Cowan's niece Terry was studying to be a special education teacher, and did her student teaching internship at Melmark between her junior and senior year. Our home was her home during the internship. When she graduated, she secured a teaching position at there, and again lived with us for a year. She kept us up-to-date on the activities and operations there, and her comments matched those of our friend at church. She said, from her observation, that we would be very pleased when Doug and Amy could move there. We could be assured that the care would be exceptional.

"When there is a question in any situation between a resident and a staff member or an aide, the resident is always 'right' no matter what happened in an incident," she said.

I agreed with that idea to a certain extent, but I realized that there could be extenuating circumstances. It gave me assurance, however, that Doug and Amy's best interests would come first. Her observations made me even more determined to continue to pursue Melmark.

In 1979, Douglas, at age seventeen, and Amy, at age twelve, moved into their new home. This did not happen without mixed feelings on my part. I was confused, apprehensive, and hurt. Why, after all these years of caring for these children, would God allow this problem that meant they had to leave our home and family? Would strangers give them the same loving care we had and treat them as if they were family?

We visited every chance we could, and it did not take long for us to realize their "new home" was not a place with which we could be totally pleased. We were required to call at least twenty-four hours before visiting to let the staff know we were coming. This did not sit well, but if that was the rule, we would abide by it. One Sunday after church we decided to travel the two hours and make an unannounced visit. When we arrived, we were told that since they did not know we were coming, we would have to wait and maybe they could arrange to bring Doug and Amy to the visitors' room for a visit.

Why would the fact that they did not know we were coming be a problem? Cowan said, "No, that is not satisfactory. We want to go to see them in their rooms." The answer was, "No, we can't allow that." Again, Cowan said, "We will go to them in their rooms, and now."

By this time they must have realized that we were not leaving without a visit, and after a long wait, we were allowed to go to visit them in their rooms. We were horrified. It was two p.m. and everyone we saw, except Doug and Amy, was still in pajamas. Doug and Amy were dressed, but we knew that was why the wait had been so long before we were allowed to see them. On subsequent visits we saw other conditions that were very bothersome.

We began to plead with God daily to open up places for them at Melmark—and soon, please.

On another visit—that was announced the day before—we were again horrified. While visiting, something drew our attention to both of their mouths, and it was evident that their teeth were not being well cared for. I could not see any separations between the teeth—a heavy build-up of plaque. Their teeth must not have been brushed for who knows how long!

The next day I called our social worker and asked if she ever made unannounced surprise visits. She said on occasion she did. I asked her if she would make one and let me know what she found. I did not tell her what we saw, or why I wanted her to make an unannounced visit. She called me the following day and said she was glad I'd asked for a surprise visit—she, too, was horrified at what she saw. She said the facility had been written up with notice that a list of things better change.

She asked why we were concerned, and I told her about the teeth. She said yes, that is one of the things she noticed, along with it being one p.m. and all residents were still in pajamas, which included Doug and Amy, and most of them were still in bed. The changes the social worker required happened for two or three months, but then we noticed things began to slip back into the same routine again.

We were getting anxious, and began to wonder if we had made the right decision to move them to this facility. But we thought we had no other choice. Doug and Amy were very responsive and interactive to stimulation when they were home with us, and also in their association with their "schooling" at the Intermediate Unit. Now we noticed they were not smiling, laughing, or responding to stimulation as they had before. It seemed they were regressing.

Looking around the room and other places we passed when going to their room, we saw there was no evidence of equipment to provide activities for stimulation. On many subsequent visits, we realized the residents were just sitting around—most with blank faces.

I began to feel that rather than this being a home away from home for Doug and Amy, it was reminding me of the institutions I had visited while I was on the board of directors for ACCESS. With each visit, we watched Doug and Amy become more and more like the other residents, sitting with blank stares, and both becoming distant and non-responsive, even to us. This did not appear to be a happy place for them, and as a matter of fact, not for any of the residents. The atmosphere had appeared to be a happier environment when we toured during our search for a suitable facility, but that was certainly not what we were witnessing now.

On one of our visits I felt so distressed that I told Cowan, "If we do not find them happier and more responsive on our next visit, they have to come back home. I cannot stand by and watch them decline, and watch the years of love and care we gave them thrown away."

We felt like we were on a rollercoaster with the situations occasionally getting better, only to watch them go backwards again.

Chapter 28

Through the years of dealing with Doug and Amy's issues, Cowan was still suffering with the chronic cluster headaches when one of the doctors he had been seeing suggested that a drier climate might help. Since Doug and Amy were no longer living in our home, and Lisa was away at college, we decided to purchase a motor home and do a three-month trial in Arizona where the humidity and barometric pressure would be lower. We enjoyed our time in Arizona, but it did not help alleviate his headaches.

Lisa was still attending East Carolina University in Greenville, North Carolina. We enjoyed trips back and forth to visit her there for four years in our home away from home. There were several other students living in our area who were also attending East Carolina. Our motor home became the mode of transportation back and forth to school, with me as chauffeur.

Since our family now had free time, we planned a trip to California with Lisa. We were now in a position to give her our undivided attention, which she truly deserved. But she was a teenager, and the thought of traveling alone with us—her Mom and Dad—for two weeks gave her concern. She asked if she could take along a friend. We told her no, but being the negotiator she was, she asked her dad, "How would you like to be cooped up with two teenagers for two weeks with no adult companionship?" Cowan and I thought about that comment, and it didn't take long for us to agree. We told her she could invite a friend.

While we were in California, a call came from Melmark. Good news! There was an opening, but only one. We would have to decide whether it would be for Doug or Amy. We had hoped we would not have to make a decision to separate them. Even though they probably did not recognize each other as brother and sister, the thought of having to choose one over the other and separating them was uncomfortable.

We discussed both of their situations with Mr. Krentel and decided that it should be Doug. He was close to eighteen and we were concerned about how much input we would be allowed to have on his behalf with the state when he reached adulthood, and we surely did not want him to be living in his existing conditions for the rest of his life. We wanted him settled in a good environment where his best interests would be paramount. We notified Melmark that Doug would be their new resident and approved the process to start.

By the time we arrived home from California, all the paperwork was ready for us to sign, and Doug moved to Melmark—The Home That Love Built. Now we were visiting two homes. What a difference in the love and care between the two homes, and what a difference between the residents' actions and responses! Doug was living with happy and active friends and caregivers who seemed to have genuine concern. Amy was living with distant and unresponsive "friends" and with "caregivers" who it seemed couldn't care less. Most importantly, his new home is a Christian home giving spiritual love and care, which Amy and Doug received when they lived in our home. At Melmark, Doug went to "church," which was held in the campus auditorium every Sunday. Every morning there was a prayer and devotion time with the residents.

I would kind of laugh sometimes when I thought about these two happenings. Doug could not possibly understand what was going on, but I certainly was happy and grateful for it. As for what he could understand, I was told, "No one knows what he may understand. He is just not able to respond." My comment, "Then, let's keep it going."

A requirement for entrance at Melmark is a full medical and dental checkup, which was done for Doug. All was well with the medical report, but the dental report was a disaster. The lack of dental care at the previous facility was evident—he had to have twelve teeth removed.

The Melmark dentist said dental care had clearly not been an important part of Doug's life. Well, that comment struck discord in me and was certainly not true. When Doug and Amy were living at home with us, they had regular dental visits, and their teeth were in good shape when they moved away. We brushed their teeth twice a day and they were under excellent dental care. The dentist said this situation could not have happened in such a short time. We called the dentist who had cared for Doug's dental needs for many years and told him what the Melmark dentist had said, which upset him. He said he would be happy to speak with this dentist and advise him that his assessment was not true.

When we told him the dentist's name, he said, "That is very interesting. I was his mentor while he was in dental training, and it would be a pleasure to advise him that the situation did happen in that short time because the teeth were in very excellent condition when Doug was in my care."

Douglas appeared to be very happy and content at Melmark and his personality bloomed. He certainly was not sitting in a chair or lying in bed in his pajamas at one or two o'clock in the afternoon, as he had been in his previous "home" environment. Rather, he was involved in music and art activities, therapeutic horse activities, field trips, and swimming using special equipment, and he was back to the hand-over-hand approach for personal hygiene care. No more plaque build-up!

There was an occasion when Doug was being bathed in a handicap tub, equipped with hoist equipment to lift him in and out of the tub, when an accident occurred. An aide was transferring Doug to his wheelchair, and the seat came off the hoist, and Doug fell to the floor. She was doing everything properly, but when she pushed the button to bring the chair up and swing it over to the wheelchair, the seat came off the equipment. We were told a screw that was supposed to stop the chair from coming off was missing.

The policy at Melmark is to notify parents immediately when anything of this nature occurs. We were called about the incident and were told that the aide would be let go. Our response was, "No, you better not let her go. It is not her fault that the equipment was defective." Our desire was not to place blame, and especially not on the aide. If there was blame, it was on Melmark's part for not keeping the equipment in safe and proper working condition. But even for that there was no blame to be given.

We inquired later and were told she had not been fired. We realized that incidents such as this could have happened even in our home, and if the incident was not from carelessness, we could find no fault. We were thanked for our patience and understanding. Now we knew what Cowan's niece Terry meant when she said, "It will be the staff member who will be at fault in any incident."

Chapter 29

On November 1, 1982, we received a call that Amy now had a place at Melmark. What a happy and joyful day that was! I was finally able to know that "all things work together for good," and I knew this was very good.

Amy went through the same medical and dental exams Douglas had. Her physical exam was also good, but again there was a problem with the dental exam. She lost eight teeth. This time the dentist did not say that Amy losing eight teeth was due to lack of good dental care. I'm sure he did not want that conversation with his mentor again.

Amy was still very fragile, weighing twelve pounds at fifteen years of age. The staff showed confidence and gentle care when handling her, and it did not prevent her from being included in the daily activities. Doug and Amy were in the same room, and we enjoyed every visit, and could go away feeling good and relieved. Very shortly, we noticed a great change in Amy's appearance of happiness and responsiveness, as we had with Doug. Our prayers had finally been answered, and seeing those changes gave us joy and contentment.

"And my God shall meet all your needs [Doug and Amy] according to His glorious riches in Christ Jesus" (Philippians. 4:19). He had fulfilled that promise through Melmark. Cowan and I wanted to show our appreciation in some way to the home and decided to become involved in volunteering there—mostly with the horse program. Douglas rode the horse in the therapeutic program, but Amy, being so delicate, was not able to sit on the horse. She rode in a pony cart pulled by a horse, still getting the therapeutic benefit of the horse's movements.

As we observed the gentle touches and the great hygiene care given there, which was so different from the previous living arrangement, we had complete confidence that our bundles of joy were in loving and caring hands. The relief from the constant concern about Doug and Amy's care, and the fact that we had no more hands-on responsibility ourselves, lifted a great burden. The heartache and frustration we had experienced with our bundles of joy through the years was now being overshadowed with this blessing of God's provision of excellent care.

Lisa graduated from college and started working. She met Brian, the man of her dreams, and we soon realized that there was going to be a wedding. The date was set and plans began for the big day in October 1990. But before we could give our permission for the marriage, we required they get genetic counseling. We truly felt that Dr. Spitz's assessment of the situation with Doug was not genetic as we had been told, but we wanted Lisa and Brian to have peace of mind that they and their children would not have to face similar trials. We felt that Brian's family should also be given that peace of mind.

The results showed that there should be no problems. This has proven to be true because years later we now have two wonderful grandchildren, both very bright, and the delight of our lives.

Preparations for the wedding started, invitations were sent out, and responses began to arrive. Family members planned to attend from many different states. Most of them had not been to Melmark, and we knew they would enjoy seeing Doug and Amy and their home. We felt it would not be advisable for Doug and Amy to attend the wedding ceremony, but we wanted them to be a part of the celebration for Lisa and Brian in some way.

A great idea came to us. Doug and Amy could "give" a wedding tea at Melmark in honor of Lisa and Brian the day before the wedding. Their friends and fellow residents at Melmark, who were at higher functioning levels, made the invitations for us to send to the family members in Doug and Amy's name. They also prepared and served the tea, and gave tours through the greenhouse, weaving room, art room, and kitchen—the areas where they did their "jobs." They also took the family on tours of Doug and Amy's room, the activity and music rooms, the swimming pool, the horse riding ring, and the auditorium. They were very proud to show off their home, and the home of their friends, Doug and Amy.

As Doug was approaching eighteen, we became concerned about what would happen to him if we were no longer around to watch out for him and his needs. We questioned what had happened at that first hernia surgery. Dr. Spitz had mentioned his concerns as to whether the blood work-up had been properly performed prior to the first surgery. Was a clotting test done on Doug's blood, and was care taken to read all the results of the blood tests?

We discussed our concerns with family, friends, doctors, and our pastor, and their advice was to consult an attorney. It seemed to them that we should at least get some expert advice. If negligence was the reason for his condition, and a lawsuit could prove it, a financial settlement could be set aside in a trust fund for his future care.

We contacted an attorney, whom we had been told had great success in winning difficult court cases. We had an interview with him and he told us he would not take the case unless he was pretty sure he could win it. So we had several more interview sessions with him, and he finally said he felt we had a good case and he would work with us. We were to give him the name and address of the hospital and the doctors' names. Of course, we couldn't remember the doctors' names, but we did give him the hospital name and address.

He began his search but quickly found that the hospital where Doug's first hernia surgery was performed had endured a fire and all records had been destroyed. He said we could continue with a lawsuit, but without records to prove what had occurred it would be a long and difficult road. He was concerned that a trial as difficult as this would be, giving testimony and being cross-examined, and opening up old wounds, would be very time consuming and difficult for us, but he was willing to continue if we still wanted to try.

We spent a great deal of time thinking and praying about what we should do, and finally decided to just let it go and trust the Lord to provide care for Douglas should it become necessary.

Chapter 30

Cowan's chronic cluster headache problem continued to haunt him. In 1994, our friends Cliff and Ginnie Johnson, who had a house at the shore, were sunning on the beach when Cliff mentioned that he hadn't seen their neighbor for a while. The gentleman, whose name was Bill, said he had been away having an operation that had given him relief from the terrible headaches with which he had suffered for many years.

Cliff had known about Bill's headaches for some time, and he was curious about the surgery. He told Bill he was interested because he had a friend who had headaches that seemed to be similar. Bill asked if he could have our phone number. He called Cowan and told him about the surgery and how it had helped him. They commiserated about the headaches and the debilitating effects they caused. Bill told Cowan he knew this doctor at the University of Pittsburgh could get rid of his pain, too. He encouraged Cowan to just give the doctor a call and at least see what he said.

It sounded encouraging, but after all the years of trying so many different suggestions to get relief with no results, Cowan felt he really didn't want to go through another procedure. Long ago he had lost hope of being without pain and had resigned himself to the fact that this would be part of his life—he just had to be tolerant and live with it, he figured. Fortunately, Bill kept after Cowan to call the doctor, and told him if he didn't, he would be calling every week until Cowan did make the call.

"I know you can get relief. Please call," Bill said.

When Cowan made the appointment, the neurosurgeon's office asked him to obtain the X-rays, MRIs, and files from all the doctors and clinics he had seen for the headaches, and to bring them to the first appointment. With so many different places to contact, this presented quite a chore, and it took a while to collect them.

When we arrived with the stack of X-rays and files, the doctor said, "If you have been to all these places, tried all these treatments, and found no relief, I am your last hope." He turned to Cowan. "Do you ever feel like banging your head against a brick wall?"

Cowan's answer: "Yes, most of the time. There are times when I don't care if I live or die. In fact, if I'd had a gun, I would have been tempted to use it."

I had lived with him through the years of his pain, and I understood why he felt this way. The doctor seemed to understand too, and he said, "You are going to be very pleased with this surgery. You will know immediately when you wake up that the headaches and suffering are gone. You will just feel different."

We were told that this particular surgery for chronic cluster headaches was the only surgery this doctor performed, and as far as he knew he was the only doctor who performed the surgery. With him being the only doctor giving this relief, there were thousands who needed him from all around the world. He said he did fifteen of these surgeries every day, five days a week.

An explanation of the intracranial surgery was a little disconcerting. There was a one percent chance Cowan would lose his hearing. The doctor would drill a small hole in the mastoid bone behind the ear to provide access to the area of the brain where the surgeon felt the problem existed.

That one percent chance of his losing his hearing was a concern to me. Wasn't being legally blind enough? We just had to trust that deafness would not occur.

The day came for the surgery. Cowan did an audio test to record his hearing level before the surgery for comparison afterward. After Cowan was rolled in for surgery, as I had done so many times through the years I anxiously waited and prayed for a successful surgery. Of some concern to me was the fact that they were going into the brain area during this surgery. As surgery was nearing closure, the surgical nurse came and gave the report that all had gone well.

She said, "The doctor said, 'Oh my ____. There's no wonder this man has headaches; it looks like scrambled eggs in here. The nerves and arteries are intertwined and in some instances have grown together. This has caused short circuits in the nerves, and that is what caused the pain.'"

She continued to say with a glimmer of amusement on her face as she watched for my response, "The nerves and arteries have been separated and (believe it or not) Teflon has been placed between them to keep them apart."

I must have had a surprised look at hearing that Teflon was used. It sounded strange to me, but if it works, who cares? The first thing Cowan said to me when he returned to his room after the surgery was exactly what the doctor had told him: "I do feel different. The headaches are gone. I haven't felt like this for years."

After fifteen years, that was the end of the cluster headaches and the medications—hallelujah! The doctor did warn him if he ever had a bad head injury to expect to need the surgery again because the Teflon could shift out of place. "You will know instantly because those terrible headaches will return," he said.

Bill found out that was true. He fell off a ladder, banged his head, and had to have the surgery again. At this point we began to wonder if Douglas had been experiencing the same headaches during the years he was banging his head and had to wear the boxing glove. Was he in the same terrible pain his Dad had experienced? If we had only known!

Chapter 31

Doug lived many happy years at Melmark. Then he started developing periodic bouts of pneumonia, aspiration, and congestive heart failure. With each episode he would be hospitalized. The back and forth trips from Melmark to the hospital continued for several months. We began to realize that these trips were not bringing healing results. I asked the nurse at if he was ever going to be free from this back and forth regimen. She said no, probably not, it would continue to be a chronic and worsening problem.

She explained that they are required to send him to the hospital each time an incident occurred. The hospital would continue to keep him only until the situation stabilized, and then they would send him back to home until the next time.

The incidents continued and the ambulance trips kept getting closer together. During one of our visits when Doug was in the hospital, the doctor asked if he could speak to us in the hall. With the doctor basically confirming what the nurse at Melmark had told us, we realized this situation was not going to get better. We asked Melmark officials if we had the right to make the decision of whether or not to continue sending Doug to the hospital. Again we were told, in their position, they had to send him, but as his guardians we could instruct them not to do so, if that was our desire.

We made that decision, and were ready to let God do his perfect will. Not long after, we received a phone call at three a.m., asking if we still did not want Doug to be sent to the hospital. We said not to send him, and that we would be there as soon as possible. When we arrived, we could see that he was not doing well, and was struggling. He was on oxygen and was very restless, fighting to take off the oxygen mask. Because the mask was strange to him, he couldn't understand that it was there to help him. We watched the struggling for some time and finally asked the nurse what would happen if the mask were removed. She said she did not know, but she had been thinking about that too.

We decided to have the oxygen mask removed, and Doug gave a sigh of relief, settled down, and seemed to be comfortable. During the next few hours our hearts were blessed by the steady stream of staff and caregivers who came by to say their good-byes to Douglas. We were touched by the sincere concern they had for the inevitable loss of their friend. At about eleven a.m., seeing that he was resting well, the nurses said we should go home and get some sleep. God was in control now, and He alone knew what would be.

At one p.m. we received a call to return, and shortly after we arrived, on March 24, 1994, God called Doug, heaven's special child, back to Him. Doug passed away peacefully. Although his passing did make me sad, at the same time my thoughts were to thank the Lord. I knew he now had a perfect body and mind. He is walking, talking, seeing, and understanding things his life on earth had denied him.

The representation of friends, neighbors, business associates, and Melmark staff and caregivers at the memorial service of celebration for Doug's life brought joy to our hearts. Our pastor had been at the church only a short time, and didn't know much about Doug and his history. He spoke with several church members and asked for their assessment of his life. I am not sure what he was told, but the sermon basically said "he did what he could do." Yes, he did what he could do even though he never spoke a word or did a deed.

I miss Doug. He was one of my bundles of joy—one of the strands of joy woven into the design of my life. I had peace in my heart knowing that he was in heaven and free from all disabilities, and that someday I would be with him again. If he could have talked with us, or in some way sent a message, I'm sure he would have said, "Hey, Mom and Dad, you should see me now. My handicaps are all gone. I'm walking. I can see Jesus. I'm talking with Jesus and singing with the angels. I am now truly fearfully and wonderfully made."

And I would finish that Bible verse by saying, "Lord, Your works are wonderful, I know that full well."

Chapter 32

Amy still resides at Melmark. She is no longer the delicate little one that everyone was afraid to hold for so many years. Lisa calls her sister "thunder thighs" because she gained weight, most of which seems to be in her legs. From being the fragile little person for so long, she is on a diet.

She is now living in a group home. This change came about as a result of some counties in Pennsylvania (Delaware County being the county of our residence) wanting to receive federal monies to help fund programs at mentally retarded residences in their respective counties. That was all well and good, but Melmark had concerns about receiving the funds, and made the decision to decline. We were told that, with the spiritual tone of their programs, they were concerned the federal government would refuse to give funding if they continued those activities. They were also concerned that if they did accept the funds, they might in the future be forced, to stop the religious activities. The powers that be at Melmark were not about to let that happen, and we were in total agreement. Faith was the founding platform of this home.

County officials informed the parents that our children would have to leave the home and move to group homes. The parents had many conversations with several county officials regarding this situation. We were finally told we had no choice other than to pay for the care at Melmark ourselves, or take our children home to live with us.

We knew we would not be able to do either of the two options. The years had gone by since Doug and Amy left home—Amy had grown to be much heavier than when she left our home, and Cowan still had the restrictions for lifting. And, we were now older, and we knew we could not physically handle caring for her.

Eventually, Melmark decided to incorporate group homes into their care program by setting them up off the main campus. They were to be run as an intermediate care facility for the mentally retarded. Fortunately, that decision was made before we had to make any decisions regarding where Amy would be living.

Amy moved to her group home on May 5, 1996. We still had concerns. A Melmark administrator ran the homes, and the care provided was the same excellent care that was given on the main campus. Amy appeared to be just as happy as she had been on the main campus. She probably did not realize there had been a change in her living arrangements. In fact, she and a particular childcare worker in her new home developed a special bond with each other.

The care at this home was on a one-on-one basis, and this particular caregiver was the person caring for Amy. She asked permission several times to take Amy home to have dinner with her family. I felt this showed her affection for Amy because it meant she had to do hand-over-hand feeding and be responsible for changing diapers, etc., which she had done at work all day long.

Melmark was okay with the arrangement as long as we gave permission, which we did. On one occasion as she was taking Amy out of bed and transferring her to the wheelchair, she and Amy both fell to the floor. As Amy fell, her face hit the footboard of the bed and she ended up in the hospital with a broken jaw. I felt sorry for the aide. She was frantic. We were notified what had happened, and that Amy was on her way to the hospital. We also were told that the aide would be let go, and again we said we would not be pleased if that happened.

The jaw had to be set and wired. Fortunately, Amy's diet was pureed food, so that was a blessing since feeding her would have been difficult otherwise. Unfortunately, soon after her jaw was wired and began to heal, a discovery was made that there had been two breaks at the time of the accident instead of just the one that was wired. At this point Amy went back into the hospital. The jaw had to be broken again and reset. My thoughts were, *my poor child, hasn't she been through enough?*

Amy does not appreciate the hand-over-hand activities that are part of her daily routine, such as brushing her teeth, washing her face, feeding herself, and so on. However, she does enjoy the attention the care aides give her—"taking" her to the "beauty salon," which is her room. She is very cooperative while they do whatever they want with her hair and paint her fingernails and toenails.

When going to visit, you might find her with every fingernail painted a different color, or sparkles in the polish, and of course the toenails have to match. As touchy as she has always been, it amazes me that she will sit for hairdos and nail painting. I think the reason she tolerates it may be the attention she gets and the comments about how cute she looks. Who knows, maybe she does understand! What woman does not love to hear flattering comments about her appearance?

At one of my visits, my eyes just about popped out of my head when I saw Amy with a head full of cornrows. She has a very thick head of hair, and I asked the aides if they knew what was going to happen when they took the cornrows out because I knew she would have a head of bushy, curly hair. Later the staff called me and said, "You were right, you should see her. We will never do that again!" It took more than a week to get the hair to settle down, even with washing and conditioning every day.

Suitable clothes for Amy are difficult to find. If I considered clothes for her age, the style was much too sophisticated for someone of her size and condition. For her birthday one year, I remembered the sparkly nail polish and thought I would see if I could find something similar. I had such a great time shopping for the sparkly polish, and even found clear makeup for her face and arms with sparkles in it. The colors that teenagers were wearing then were bright chartreuse, hot pink and bright turquoise. I found shorts and tops in those colors and the sparkling polish to match.

One day Amy was dressed in the bright clothes with polished fingernails and toenails and the clear glittery makeup on, she had a seizure and was taken to the hospital. An aide from Melmark always goes to the hospital with a resident, and an aide stays twenty-four hours, rotating shifts. The aides feed the patient and take care of other needs while in the hospital. It works best for the aides to be there because they are familiar with the residents and their habits, and it relieves the nurses who do not have the time it takes to feed them. On this particular occasion, the aide said word traveled around the hospital about a resident from Melmark, who most likely does not have a clue as to what is going on, but you should see her fingernails, toenails, face, and arms.

The reported result for the seizure was that her medication needed to be changed. Seizure medication changes are a normal occurrence. As Amy grew and/or put on weight, the doses needed to be increased to keep the seizures under control.

One day while Amy was eating lunch, she aspirated food into her lungs. She apparently did not know how to cough as the food was going down the wrong way to keep it out of her lungs, so she ended up choking. She was taken to the hospital for observation. The aspiration must have been very uncomfortable because after that incident, she refused to eat. The doctor said she was probably afraid it would hurt again. She was put on an IV for nourishment until she would begin eating again.

But Amy continued to refuse food. Many days went by with her still not eating. We watched as she became weaker and weaker, and as she finally went into a semi-comatose state. The aides who went to the hospital to stay with her and the hospital staff tried many different ways to encourage her to eat, with no success. We were finally asked to make a very difficult decision: permission to install a feeding tube. The thought of her needing a feeding tube had not entered my mind. Our first reaction was not to do it because of the long-term ramifications we felt it might bring. But then the doctors told us she was losing strength, and they felt if she could get her strength back she might start eating again, and the feeding tube could provide that opportunity.

Amy was now well past the age of twenty-one, and our concern was that if the feeding tube did not give her strength and she still refused to eat, would we legally have the right to make the decision to have the feeding tube removed at some future time? We watched and waited for days for her to start eating or for some change, but the situation did not change. We realized something had to be done because she could not live without food.

Again we felt trapped in a catch twenty-two situation. The concerns we had about the feeding tube were due to stories we had seen in the news about feeding tube situations ending up in court battles between the medical community and the patient's family. We were told that the feeding tube would not have to be permanent, and it could be removed within seconds when it was no longer needed. But who makes the decision as to when it would not be needed? This was an important decision, and it caused us sleepless nights.

We asked Lisa, our critical care nurse daughter, to help us decide. We knew she had dealt with these kinds of situations at the hospital, and we trusted her advice. She was in agreement with the doctors that the feeding tube would probably give Amy's body the strength she needed to recover, and the possibility of starting to eat again. She felt we really did not have any other choice. If we did not agree, Amy would starve to death. We knew we could not let that happen.

We were again praying for guidance and the answer to our dilemma. We also kept the Internet busy for a couple days, sending e-mails to family and friends around the country, asking for prayer on Amy's behalf and for the Lord to help us know what to do about this difficult decision. Assurance finally came that the feeding tube was necessary, and we approved the surgery.

Lisa and the doctors were correct. Amy did regain strength, started eating, and soon was able to return home to Melmark. The doctors convinced us to leave the feeding tube in—just in case that situation occurred again—so she would not have to go through surgery again.

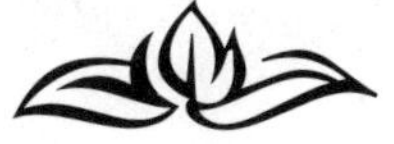

Chapter 33

I must confess that at times as I faced difficult and heart-breaking situations with Doug and Amy, I felt like the teacup in the antique shop in England that I mentioned in the beginning of this journey:

> "Stop it! Stop it!"
> "Leave me alone."
> "I'm getting dizzy."
> "I'm burning up."

I begged. I pleaded. But all the time, God was just saying, "Not now. Not yet." I know that—like the teacup—at times I have been impatient when prayers were not answered immediately, or in the way I wanted them to be answered.

I know prayers are answered in three ways: Yes—things happen as I have asked. No—the request is never granted because God knows what I asked was not the best. Not now—the answer may come much later and even in a different way than I had in mind. But, I thank God for answering my prayers in the ways He has. I know that, through it all, He has given constant, abiding love.

As the quiet voice, I heard many times told me, He never left or forsook me. He helped me through the struggles and trials. I also cannot say that there were not times when, for a fleeting moment, I thought, *why?* And *is this really the "best" for me?* I especially doubted when others asked the "why" questions. But my thoughts would return, saying, *Why not me? Yes, why not me? I am God's to use as He needs and chooses, and if it is His will, it should give me a sense of pride that He knows I am capable of doing the job.* Through it all, I saw that the trials I thought were going to destroy me became the building blocks that brought joy to my life. As the master said to the teacup, might it be that God could say to me, "You are what I had in mind when I first began with you, and now you can be useful to me."

There must have been a reason He needed me to be the mother of two of heaven's very special children. Joy can be defined as the emotion of great delight or happiness caused by something exceptionally good. My journey through the years with Doug, Amy, and Lisa has certainly been ones of "great delight and happiness" even though there were times of sorrow, sadness, and frustration. I consider those trials, sorrows, and sad times "something exceptionally good," because they brought "delight and happiness" that far overshadowed the sorrow, sadness, and frustration.

Up to this point in my journey I have written mainly about Douglas, Lisa, and Amy. But, as the commentator, Paul Harvey said, "And now the rest of the story." I have another joy that was added to my bundle: my husband, Cowan, who has been my partner and travel companion on the journey. As I placed my hand in his hand during our wedding ceremony, I made a lifelong commitment, and I promised to love and cherish him through joy and sorrow, in sickness and in health, for better or worse, till death parts us. We have worked together through the many issues of our lives, and in all of these, the love and cherishing we have felt for each other is what has helped to make our marriage strong and happy.

It was especially difficult for Cowan to travel the journey while he was experiencing his own health and physical problems—back surgery, cluster headaches, brain surgery, and macular degeneration bringing legal blindness—all while we were dealing with the trials in Doug and Amy's lives. It has been just as stressful for me to watch and help him through those times as it was to deal with the situations with Doug and Amy. It would be difficult to know how to express my appreciation for the support, understanding, and help he has given me.

Chapter 34

In the fall of October 1999, Cowan and I were on our way to Toledo to visit our families. We were not very far into the trip when Cowan started shaking with chills and at the same time said he felt like he was burning up. When we arrived at the motel where we planned to spend the night, I asked if we should go the hospital and he said no, that he would probably be okay once he got into bed and got a good night's sleep.

It was a miserable night for both of us. We got no sleep. He shook so violently that I was surprised he did not walk the bed across the floor. We continued on to Toledo the next morning with his chills, shaking, and burning feeling continuing. When we arrived at his sister's, she encouraged him to go to the hospital.

Our home was on a wooded lot. We had always dreamed of such a home. Every morning we watched a herd of fourteen deer pass by just inside the edge of the woods, and then in the evening we watched them return in the opposite direction. We had heard on the news that the tick population was bad that year, and to be cautious if you lived in a wooded area. The news reports had given the symptoms to watch for: chills, trembling, and burning sensations. Since deer are good hosts for ticks, the woods are a perfect breeding ground. Cowan was experiencing all the symptoms that accompany Lyme disease. We told the doctors we thought it might be that.

Their response was that Lyme disease could not be the problem. However, they had no clue what the problem was. He was given a shot to calm his system, and they sent him on his way. Even though the doctors at the hospital in Toledo said Lyme disease could not be what he was experiencing, we were still so sure that the symptoms mentioned on the news matched what Cowan had experienced, that when we returned home we made an appointment with our doctor for a checkup. The look on our doctor's face, and his gasp when he examined Cowan was priceless.

Cowan had five bulls-eyes on his back and one under his arm.

The doctor said, "You certainly have been bitten by ticks. By the time the bulls-eyes show up like this; the ticks are gone and have left havoc behind. You now have Lyme disease, and once you have it you will always have it."

He started Cowan on an antibiotic treatment. He said that Lyme disease could present lifelong debilitating effects in many areas of the body.

A friend who was being treated for Lyme disease gave Cowan a booklet published by the Lyme Disease Association with information on the subject. The booklet included a list of about one hundred ways the body can be affected, and Cowan has experienced many of them: heart attack, chronic backaches, headaches, poor balance, difficulty walking, stroke symptoms, acid reflux, elevated blood pressure, carpal tunnel in both hands requiring surgery, chronic fatigue syndrome, and joint pain and stiffness. These medical conditions have all occurred since the tick incident.

On May 2, 2000, another detour was added to our journey. I was on phone-answering duty at work and received a call from our friend Angelo telling me that Cowan was in an ambulance on the way to the hospital. Cowan and I managed a rental listing, and he and Angie were getting it ready for new tenants. When Angie called me, he said he did not think it was too serious, but I probably should get to the hospital as soon as possible.

Angie had been a paramedic, and I knew he knew more than he was telling me. He told me Cowan was being taken to a hospital that was about a three-minute trip from where they were working. I found someone to take over the phone duty and left on a frantic drive. I could feel, just from his tone of voice and the way he stated the situation, that Angie was not telling me the whole story. The drive from my office to the hospital was going to take about twenty to twenty-five minutes.

During that frantic drive, I thought that if the situation were very serious he would probably be in the operating room by the time I arrived—or even worse! I was stopped for a stoplight about one or two minutes from the hospital and watched an ambulance coming from the direction of our friend's house as it turned toward the hospital. I thought *that can't be Cowan in there. With the short distance they had to travel, they should have been in the emergency room long ago.*

When I arrived at the emergency room I found the doctors and nurses frantically working with Cowan. I was told he had just arrived. *So that was him in that ambulance I saw at the stop light!* The news was not good. He had a heart attack. I was taken into the room where they were in the process of preparing him to do a super clot-buster procedure. I was asked to sign forms giving permission. I sat in the room watching as they were preparing Cowan for the surgery. I heard the doctor ask him, "Is there anything you want to tell your wife?" and I heard Cowan say, "Tell her I love her."

I was beginning to realize the seriousness of the situation because the tone of the doctor's voice told me he really meant, "Is there anything you want me to tell your wife since you may be leaving this world?" I realized something had to be done to take care of Cowan, but it dawned on me that the procedure they were preparing to do was probably not good. Clot-busting probably meant pressure would be put on his arteries—and what would that do to his eyes?

I asked them to wait and told the cardiologist about the bleeding retinas Cowan had experienced, causing legal blindness.

He said, "Let me have those papers back, we can't do this procedure," and he tore up the papers I had just signed.

I asked him to call his ophthalmologist and see what he thought. He called and the answer was, "Absolutely not! He would have serious hemorrhaging and probably end up totally blind."

The cardiologist said, "If we can't do the clot-buster procedure, there is nothing we can do in this hospital. We need to send him to another hospital where intervention angioplasty can be done."

He called another hospital and told the cardiologist there what the situation was. He was put back in the ambulance, I was put in the front seat, and off we went for a twenty-minute ride to the other hospital.

On the way the ambulance driver told me the reason it had taken so long to get him from our friend's home to the first hospital was that they had lost him three times, and had to stop each time to bring him back. With that bit of news, and hearing what was going on behind me, I was just about to have a heart attack myself. With all the scenarios, I had envisioned while driving from work to the hospital still going through my mind, and now this, I began to pray, and pray hard.

My mind had so many thoughts going through it that I'm not sure my jumbled prayers were making any sense to the Lord, but He knew what was on my heart. He told us to ask, and it would be given. I was not only asking, but I was begging. I knew that God was in control of this situation, as He had been with Doug and Amy so many times. He had brought them through some very serious and difficult times, and I knew He could do the same for Cowan. I finally said to myself, *be still my heart, and let God's will be done.*

When we arrived at the second hospital, the cardiologist was waiting for us at the emergency entrance. He asked Cowan, "On a scale from one to ten, how bad is the pain?"

"Eleven," Cowan said.

The doctor said, "Great," and motioning to the paramedics, said, "Get him into the operating room now."

Great! I thought. *What can he mean—a pain level higher than on the doctor's scale is great?* I found my way to the waiting room and called Lisa. She lives in Wilmington, Delaware, and the drive would take her about an hour to make the trip to the hospital. I felt sorry for her getting that kind of news on that particular day, because it was Brian's birthday. I'm sure she had something special planned to celebrate. One thing is sure: Cowan will never forget the date of his son-in-law Brian's birthday.

Lisa came to sit with me. And of course as a critical care nurse she wanted to hear the doctor's report and see for herself that he was okay. The doctor came to the waiting room to bring me up to date on the situation. It was over; Cowan's primary heart artery had been totally blocked and another one was 70 percent blocked. Intervention angioplasty was performed to clear the arteries, and two stints were put into keep them open.

The doctor said, "He is looking good, and is definitely more comfortable. I could tell by the look on your face that you were concerned when I said 'great' at the pain level being eleven. I wanted to explain why, but I knew we had to get to work immediately, because I knew he did not have much time left, in fact, he only had about ten minutes to live."

I was relieved that the surgery was over but at the same time I had an anxious feeling at hearing that he had been so close to death, again. We were grateful for all who had been the Lord's helpers during the hour or so before the surgery.

Cowan was feeling so well that five days after the surgery; he and I delivered fruit baskets to show our thanks and appreciation to the first hospital emergency room, the cardiologist there, the ambulance crew, and the cardiologist who performed the surgery.

The doctor must have truly believed that ten minutes was all the time Cowan had left to live, because when we delivered the fruit basket to his office his nurse said, "You must be the miracle man we've been hearing about. The doctor was so sure that you had such a short time to live that he sent letters of commendation to the other hospital administration, their emergency room staff, the cardiologist, and the ambulance crew, thanking them for not trying to be heroes. If they had, Cowan would have died."

Her comments reminded me of the time Amy was in the hospital and recovered from a coma and the doctor said, "It's just not her time; there must be something for her to do." As with Amy, the Lord was not ready for Cowan yet. There had to be something left for him to do. I definitely knew one thing he had to do—continue to be my husband.

An interesting aside to this situation is that if Cowan had been at our home, instead of at our friend's, when this happened, he probably would not have lived. It would have taken the ambulance about ten minutes to get to our home, and our home was about ten minutes from the hospital. When you add up those times, the ambulance could not have gotten to him and then to the hospital before the three "death" incidents occurred. In addition, the hospital where he would have been taken did not do the angioplasty surgery either, and he would have been sent twenty-five miles from there to the very hospital where the surgery had been performed. We are thankful that God is in control of all that happens in our lives. He placed Cowan where the timing worked.

In 2007, other Lyme disease effects began to surface in Cowan, causing serious problems with his balance and difficulty walking. He sought a neurosurgeon's advice and help. Tests were ordered, and it was determined that the balance and walking problems could be because Cowan had normal pressure hydrocephalus, and a VJ shunt was needed. Of course, we already knew about the shunt since Amy had had one implanted years earlier. We knew it helped relieve the normal pressure hydrocephalus for her. But the shunt did not put an end to the balance problem for Cowan—in fact, his balance problem continued to worsen and he had to start using a cane to give him confidence and stability.

Then Cowan began to have even more difficulty with balance and walking, and he occasionally had falling incidents. In May 2010, in about a three-week span of time, he went from a cane to using a walker to a seated Rollator walker, and then a wheelchair as he was not able to stand or bear weight on his feet.

Cowan's neurosurgeon called for an MRI. It revealed a collapsed spinal column, which he said was preventing messages from getting from the brain to the lower extremities of his body. The decision was made to do thoracic laminectomy surgery and open up the spinal column. Cowan spent four weeks in a physical rehabilitation hospital, where he was basically taught to walk again. The doctor was hopeful the surgery would allow Cowan to walk without a cane, but that has not yet happened. We do praise God that Cowan is walking, even if it is with a cane.

Chapter 35

I share the story of life's journey with my bundles of joy with an attitude of praise and thanks to God. He gave Doug, Lisa, Amy, and Cowan to me, and even though there have been difficult and frustrating roads to travel with them, they have brought much joy into my life.

The following are some of the joys that are dear to me—the ones God and I have been through together as He and I have walked the roads of joy, love, laughter, trial, and discouragement:

- Joy of answered prayer.
- Joy of knowing peace that passes all understanding.
- Joy of knowing and feeling God's constant and abiding love.
- Joy of finding patience through trials.
- Joy of knowing I could trust the Lord to know what is best.
- Joy of strength from the Lord to accomplish all that had to be done.
- Joy of the knowledge that my life may have been helpful to others.
- Joy of firsthand knowledge that the Lord will never allow burdens that He will not also help to carry

Thinking back to the question I was asked in the beginning of my story, "How do you feel toward God because of the trials He has allowed into your life?" I thank Him because I know He has walked with me through the trials, and has given me the strength I needed to handle them. On an occasion, I have said that I am going to be the first in line when I get to heaven to ask the "why" questions. But then I realized that those questions will no longer be important. They will not matter. I probably will not even remember the times of trial. What I do hope to hear is, "Well done good and faithful servant," and from Douglas and Amy, "Thank you, Mom, for loving and caring for us."

The words of the song, **Thank You Lord**, written by Dan Burgess, shares my feelings and answer the "How do you feel toward God?" questions.

Thank you, Lord,
for the trials that come my way.
In that way I could grow each day
as I let you lead,
And I thank you, Lord,
for the patience those trials bring.
In that process of growing,
I have learned to care.

But it goes against the way I am
to put my human nature down
and let the Spirit take control of all I do.

'Cause when those trials come,
my human nature shouts the things to do,
and God's soft prompting can be easily ignored.

I thank you, Lord,
with each trial I feel inside,
that you're there to help,
lead and guide me away from wrong.
'Cause you promised, Lord,
that with every testing
that your way of escaping is easier to bear.

But it goes against the way
I am to put my human nature down
and let the Spirit take control of all I do.

'Cause when those trials come,
my human nature shouts the thing to do;
and God's soft prompting
can be easily ignored.

I thank you, Lord,
For the victory that growing brings.
In surrender of everything,
life is so worthwhile.
And I thank you, Lord,
that when everything's put in place,
out in front I can see your face,
and it's there you belong.